D0556486

# NEEM

## India's Miraculous Healing Plant

## ELLEN NORTEN

edited by Jean Pütz
with Kordula Werner and
Deborah Straw

Healing Arts Press
Rochester, Vermont

Healing Arts Press
One Park Street
Rochester, Vermont 05767
www.InnerTraditions.com

Healing Arts Press is a division of Inner Traditions International

First English language edition published by Inner Traditions International
Translation copyright © 2000 by Inner Traditions International
Copyright © 1996 by vgs verlagsgesellschaft, Köln

All rights reserved. No part of this book may be reproduced or utilized in any form or by any means, electronic or mechanical, including photocopying, recording, or by any information storage and retrieval system, without permission in writing from the publisher.

*Note to the reader: This book is intended as an informational guide. The remedies, approaches, and techniques described herein are meant to supplement, and not to be a substitute for, professional medical care or treatment. They should not be used to treat a serious ailment without prior consultation with a qualified health care professional.*

**Library of Congress Cataloging-in-Publication Data**

Norten, Ellen.
      [Wunderbaum Neem. English]
      Neem : India's miraculous healing plant / Ellen Norten.—1st English
language ed.
            p.          cm.
      Includes bibliographical references.
      ISBN 978-0-89281-837-2 (alk. paper)
      1. Neem—Therapeutic use. 2. Neem products—Therapeutic use. 3. Neem.
I. Title.

RM666.N34 N65513 1999
615'.32377—dc21

                                                            99-049948

Printed and bound in the United States

10 9 8 7 6 5 4 3 2

This book was typeset in ItalianElectric

# CONTENTS

# INTRODUCTION

## NEEM—AN OMNIPOTENT TREE

At first glance you might mistake the tropical neem tree for a domestic plant. Its leaves are feathered, and the entire tree resembles an ash tree. However, you might not run into the neem tree in your latitude since it is extremely sensitive to cold. It would only survive the peak of summer outside. Even in greenhouses, it is a rare guest. Because it does not seem particularly exotic, other, more impressive trees are exhibited there. This surely is one of the reasons why the neem tree is little known in the United States; however, this is changing.

Of course, the origins of this tropical tree lie in a hot country. The neem tree comes from Myanmar (Burma) and India. It has always been honored there as a health provider for plants, animals, and humans. The word *neem* comes from Sanskrit, the origin of all Indo-European languages, and translates into "the healer and illness reliever." Around 1500 B.C. this tree was mentioned in this context in religious writings.

Today the neem tree continues to play an important role in

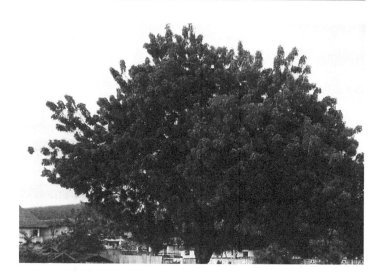

The neem tree—provider of health for humans and plants. At first glance, because of its feathered leaves, it looks like an ash tree.

Indian healing and cosmetics. In some places it is even referred to as the "village pharmacy"—rightly so, since many of the ancient recipes have been verified by scientific methods.

In regard to plant protection, the applications of neem seeds and leaves have been researched by many scientists. These experiments showed that plants treated with neem withstood many parasites: plant eaters and parasites such as caterpillars, and many types of lice and beetles can be effectively controlled with neem. More than two hundred types of insects as well as a number of mites, worms, fungi, bacteria, and even some viruses react to the ingredients in neem.

These organisms are by no means killed right away: insects, for example, turn "lazy"; they stop eating and procreating, and they no longer lay eggs. They oftentimes simply get stuck in one stage of development. Even though they are still alive, they no longer cause any damage. They die after about one to three weeks. During this time, they can serve as a "fresh" source of food for some useful insects. Birds, too, will have an easy time picking up neem-treated caterpillars.

Apart from neem not being toxic to humans, the fact that it is not harmful to the environment is another important advantage over synthetic chemical pesticides with the so-called knock-down effect. This means that after the use of a chemical shock the pests, and with them, of course, the useful insects, fall from the plants all at once.

For Indians, the neem tree is a part of daily life. As children, they learn to appreciate the advantages of this tree. Mosquito bites, for example, as well as other skin wounds are treated by applying neem leaves or neem extracts. For treatment of fever and stomach or intestinal problems, even for malaria and viral infections, strong neem teas are used. Lice, scabies, mites, and fleas are washed away with a watered-down solution of neem seeds or with prepared neem shampoos. Soaps, toothpaste, facial lotions, and nail oils contain neem extracts for cleansing and care. Neem disinfects, relieves inflammations, and lowers fevers.

It is thus no surprise that the Indians treat this plant with respect and truly honor it. Faithful Hindus on New Year's Day even bathe in water into which they have dipped neem branches. This is supposed to serve as a good omen for the coming year.

Aside from its use in medicine, cosmetics, and pesticides, neem also has a technical use: neem oil, like other plant oils, is commercially used as lamp oil and as grease.

The neem tree belongs to the family of the mahogany plants, the Meliaceae. However, its wood is by no means red; rather, it exhibits a light brown to yellowish color. The trees are evergreen but may shed a part of or even all their leaves under extreme climatic conditions, such as a lengthy drought. The single pinna (divisions of a featherlike leaf) are about two centimeters long, are light to dark green, and have a wider middle part. The sides are rigid. There are about ten leaves on one stem; they form a sort of fan that is generally shed as a whole. Botanical guides speak of "feathered" leaves, referring to the entire fan formation.

Neem leaves contain a multitude of active ingredients that are used in medicine and cosmetics as well as in plant protection. The leaves have a slightly base or alkaline character. They are, chemically speaking, the opposite of acidic. The shed leaves can contribute to neutralizing acidic ground.

Under dry, hot conditions, neem trees grow extremely quickly. The trees blossom for the first time after about three to five years. The blossoms are white, somewhat similar to a lilac's, but they are more delicate and are not as close to one another. The neem petals are either male or heterogeneous, meaning that they have both male and female flower parts or pistils. Their slightly aromatic scent attracts insects for pollination. The honey of bees that collect pollen almost exclusively from neem flowers is a special delicacy.

After the neem tree blossoms, small fruits form that, much like the leaves, hang off the branches from small stems. The fruits grow to the size and shape of olives. At first, they are a similar color to the leaves. Once they ripen, they turn yellow and soften, at which time they can be harvested. After some time, they fall off the tree by themselves.

The fruits have a good-tasting, sweet-sour flavor that, unfortunately, is not easily separated from the core and is only palatable in its completely ripe stage. Thus, they cannot always be eaten like cherries, by simply spitting out the pit. If, when eating these fruits, you hit the core, the enjoyable taste is over. The seeds taste so bitter that even the most bitter medicine tastes good in comparison—even though the seeds are in no way toxic. Only people experienced in eating the fruit are able to fully enjoy it. Most others will want to spit it out immediately.

## A TREE TRAVELS THE WORLD

At the moment, about eighteen million neem trees are growing in India, and the trees have spread throughout almost all of Southeast Asia. While in India and neighboring countries, for example, Myanmar (Burma), the neem tree grows naturally, it

The qualities of the neem tree are appreciated in many countries—partly as a desired provider of refuge from the tropical sun.

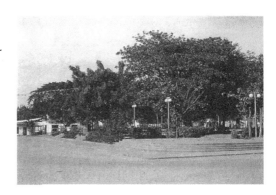

was imported to all other hot countries. It first reached West Africa via ship when humans learned to value this graceful tree, also used as firewood. Neem trees even grow in desert climates.

In hot African countries, the neem tree has become a desired plant. Niger, Nigeria, Ghana, and East African countries, as well, started to plant these trees to add green to their cities and parks. In these parts of the world, where the temperatures rise to intolerable levels, shade is a priceless commodity. In East Africa, in Sudan, in Somalia or Mauritius, the neem tree is quite common. Today almost fifty thousand neem trees provide shade for the two million Muslim pilgrims that visit Mecca in Saudi Arabia each year. The trees relieve some of the pains of the *hadsch*, the pilgrimage.

In this century, neem trees reached North and South America. In Nicaragua, Honduras, Cuba, and the Dominican Republic, the neem tree is planted on a grand scale. Venezuela is in the process of establishing the neem tree. In North America as well as in Europe, it is generally too cold for the neem tree. A few trees do grow in Florida, and a few small experimental plantations also exist in the southern United States.

## QUICKLY GROWN

Neem trees grow quickly and develop to impressive heights: they can grow to be thirty meters tall and their crown can

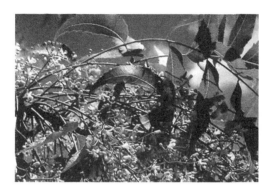

Neem trees develop quickly: after only three years, the first white blossoms start to appear between the feathered leaves.

extend to twenty meters. The trunk circumference reaches about 2.5 meters. The roots of these trees penetrate far into the ground. Under favorable conditions, neem trees are able to procreate through their roots.

The trees can live with temperatures of up to fifty degrees Celsius (in the shade) and near the equator can grow up to an elevation of 1,000 meters. They love rain. They feel most comfortable with an average yearly rainfall of 400 to 1,200 millimeters. Neem trees can grow even on dry ground that is poor in nutrients. Because the fallen leaves with their slightly base pH value of 8.2 neutralize the earth, they can exist even in acidic areas.

Neem trees can grow rather old: there are many that are at least one hundred years old. Rare, however, are those that have passed a second century.

Even though the neem tree bears its first fruits in three to five years, it reaches its maximal fruit capacity after about ten years. Then it can produce up to fifty kilograms, in extreme cases up to 150 kilograms, of fruit per year. The average harvest lies at around twenty to thirty kilograms, depending on the tree's age.

For effective plant protection using neem, a farmer for one hectare of land needs about one hundred kilograms of fruit, which corresponds to about ten kilograms of seeds. Because spraying with neem (depending on the pest) should be repeated every two to four weeks, the harvest from one tree does not quite

At first the olivelike neem fruits are light green like the leaves. The flesh of the older, yellow fruits can only be separated from the core when the fruit is completely ripe.

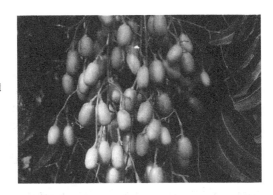

suffice for one hectare per year. Thus, a farmer should have at least four or five neem trees on his property.

Since neem trees by no means have to grow on plantations, they hardly take away from the fields of those farmers that decide to use their fruits for the protection of their crops. By planting neem, the farmer can add some green to the sides of his fields or his roads as well as his yard. He will have enough neem seeds for the protection of his crops as well as for medical uses. For commercial uses, the trees, of course, have to be grown on plantations. The economic rationale for neem plantations is most often a sound one since neem products are generally well paid for.

## HARMLESS FOR HUMANS

With the development and rapid spread of synthetic insecticides, natural pest control has been pushed more and more into the background. Maybe you still know recipes that used to be popular, such as tobacco broth or nettle extract, which today are experiencing a renaissance among environmentally minded people and are used, for example, against plant lice.

The knowledge of the usefulness of certain types of chrysanthemums for plant protection stretches back to Persian times. Two thousand four hundred years ago the Persians obtained insecticide ingredients from the chrysanthemum blossoms, the so-called pyrethrin. Today we have access to ready-made pyrethrum extracts from agricultural chrysanthemum plantations.

Over the decades, with the usage of synthetic insecticides in agriculture, forests, vineyards, and private gardens, serious consequences have developed for humans and the environment. The long-term effects of the original chemical, especially of highly chlorinated products in the environment, are often enormous. In the meantime, the products can reach the groundwater with the rain or remain as residues in the plants, and by means of the food chain, reach other living organisms. These toxic residues collect especially in the fat tissue of animals—and finally also in humans.

An ideal natural insecticide should have no undesired side effects in its production or application. It should be nontoxic to humans and quickly break down into natural substances. However, in spite of continual improvements, many of the insecticides used today only partially fulfill these conditions.

Neem ingredients bear no resemblance to such synthetic insecticides since they contain no toxic chlorine combinations. They are composed merely of carbon, hydrogen, and oxygen and are decomposed in the outdoors within a few days. Because the metabolism of humans and other vertebrates is so fundamentally different from that of insects, neem is extremely toxic to insects, but not to the higher orders of animals. This fact is confirmed through observations in nature as well as scientific studies.

Some birds and bats, for example, live off the fruits of the neem tree. In some areas, such as the Accra plains in Ghana, neem, due to lack of alternative food sources, has become the only food source for these animals. However, no changes among these animals are known.

Indians have protected their grain reserves for centuries using neem leaves or neem oil. Generations of humans have, along with their daily nutrition, taken a dose of neem, which seems to have had no negative consequences.

Initial testing on rats finds no changes in the blood of the animals after external applications of neem extracts. Moreover, studies of neem oil toxicology conducted in Germany using hand-picked, select seeds did not produce negative results. The dosage for these scientific studies, five grams of neem oil per kilogram of body weight, was mixed into the food of rats and rabbits.

A quick test for finding mutated and possibly carcinogenic characteristics of substances is the so-called Ames test, named after American biochemist Bruce N. Ames. Because of its comparatively simple experimental structure, the test has become part of a standard procedure to test for mutations. Because 90 percent of all mutation-causing substances can also act as carcinogens among higher organisms including humans, this test provides direct information about the carcinogenic effects of a substance.

The substances are tested using a bacteria, *Salmonella typhimurium*, that has a high absorption capacity for various substances. Furthermore, the bacteria is equipped with a defect repair mechanism of its gene material so that even minute mutational effects can be traced. For neem extracts as well as neem oil, no mutational effects were found using the Ames test.

In contrast to these results, however, are reports from West Africa about kidney damage that occurred after the consumption of highly concentrated neem tea extracts. Furthermore, there are records of serious illnesses, even deaths, among children in Malaysia.

Another scientific study more closely investigated the custom of some countries to feed neem oil to small children and confirmed the existence of toxic effects: if children under four years of age consume between five and thirty milliliters of neem oil per day, symptoms occur that resemble the so-called Reye's syndrome: the brain, liver, and other internal organs start to swell.

It is possible that fungi-infected seeds were the cause of such threatening illnesses. The substances produced by fungi, or mycotoxins, are often toxic to humans and cause similar illnesses.

Until the causes for the appearance of illnesses and changes are explained, the internal use of neem oil and neem extracts must be avoided. However, nothing stands in the way of the external applications of neem. Medical and cosmetic neem products as well as dental hygiene products enrich our lives, and I can recommend their use without hesitation.

## Neem is not Neem is not Neem

Even though neem trees grow only in Earth's hottest countries, some trees do live under less than ideal conditions. While in desert regions they hardly catch a drop of rain throughout the year, neem trees in parts of India experience the heavy rainfalls of the monsoon season year after year. Temperatures, length of daylight, changes between lightness and darkness, elevation, and quality of the soil also differ in the various habitats of the tree. This is one of the reasons why the active ingredients in neem significantly vary in their composition according to the plant's origin—even though the trees may not exhibit significant external differences.

Neem trees also differ from one another in a second regard: scientific studies show that they are by no means genetically identical. A Venezuelan, a Sudanese, and an Indian neem tree do not necessarily contain the same hereditary characteristics, even though they all are the same type of plant. The differences of the genes is also reflected in the composition of active ingredients of the neem. Some neem trees are better suited for medical applications, while others would be especially effective to use for plant protection.

The smell of the seeds, the oil, and the leaves also varies depending on the genetic variation. In the past several years, scientists have searched specifically for especially effective neem trees and types of neem; they were successful in their quest. In the Philippines, the so-called super neem, or giant neem (*Azadirachta excelsa*), surpasses all types of neem known so far in height, size of fruits, and potency of active ingredients. Unfortunately, only about ten of these spectacular trees—which grew to be more than fifty meters high—remain. Today, there is a concerted effort to plant more of these "super neems" in Thailand.

But other types of neem trees also show their effectiveness. All neem trees are suited to recultivate dried-up land. In principle, any neem tree can be used for human purposes, with some types being a little more efficacious than others.

## A Tree Grows In The Desert

For people living in the extremely hot regions of our earth, the neem tree plays an important role in the recultivation of arid land. There are few plants that are as tolerant to heat and as undemanding as the tropical neem tree. With its deep reaching roots, it is equipped to anchor earth threatened by erosion.

Bare ground almost always poses a threat to people: wind and rain can wash away fertile soil, leaving sandy ground behind that, depending on location, allows for little or no cultivation of plants. One of the problems with the deforestation of the tropical rain forests is not only the loss of millennia old vegetation and the often unique types of plants and animals, but also the loss of important nutrients and the earth's fertility.

After deforestation, a thin layer of fertile soil remains, which generally is usable for agriculture. The plants, however, demand so many nutrients that they exhaust soil not equipped for intensive agricultural work. Left behind are infertile plains that are now exposed to wind and rain.

On such soil, the native plants of the rain forest cannot start to grow. The land first needs to be recultivated; the ground needs to be held in place and enriched with nutrients. In such situations the neem tree can play the role of a pioneer. Because the tree grows extremely rapidly, in the extreme heat it is soon able to provide shade under which more plants can start to grow.

Unfortunately, the neem tree is not yet used for the recultivation of the barren areas of the rain forests. As the forests seem to be unlimited, deforestation continues. The farmers can always find new, freshly deforested areas when the yields on the cultivated fields decrease.

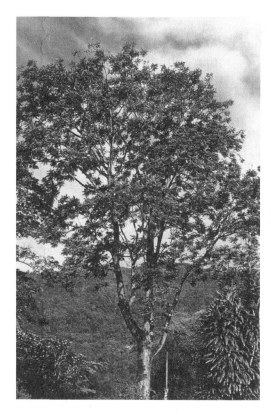

The giant neem (*Azadirachta excelsa*) surpasses all other types of neem, not only in terms of the size of the tree and its fruits, but also in the effectiveness of its ingredients.

In other areas on Earth, new areas are not always as easy to find: the Sahara is expanding to the north as well as to the south. Starvation and poverty are the result of the increasing desertification. People in desperate need of firewood cut down the existing plants to have fire to cook with.

In such desert areas, the neem tree has already come into play. Often development aid projects initiate the planting of neem trees. In Germany, for example, the GTZ, the Society for Technical Cooperation, and the Friedrich-Naumann Foundation support and plan projects such as these. On an international level the UNIDO and the UNEP, development aid and environmental organizations of the United Nations, use the neem tree and its beneficial characteristics in recultivation efforts.

Once the neem trees are planted, a real service has been provided: they make agriculture possible in many areas, and more accessible firewood can eventually be obtained from the rapidly growing trees.

Surprisingly, the use of neem as a pesticide is not known in those countries where neem grows naturally. In some Southeast Asian countries, synthetic chemical insecticides are used in great quantities even though neem trees are available in sufficient numbers. Even though the people here have known this tree for centuries and take advantage of its medicinal qualities, its application for plant protection is new to them.

This may be surprising at first glance, but neem research in the area of pesticides began only forty years ago. In 1959 Heinrich Schmutterer observed a surprising phenomenon in the Sudan: an invading swarm of grasshoppers had eaten up all the green vegetation. However, in the bare landscape, some trees remained standing with all their leaves intact. These were, of course, the neem trees. Heinrich Schmutterer at that moment may have grasped what incredible possibilities this tree could offer in the area of plant protection. This finding marked the birth of research on neem as a biological insecticide.

In the past forty years, researchers from around the world have gathered an immense amount of knowledge in this area. Thousands of scientific publications document the extensive research that has by no means yet been concluded but is expanding on a daily basis. Because the research is concentrated mainly in the United States and in other industrialized nations, the results are largely unknown among populations in the developing countries. It is thus the goal of some projects to transfer this knowledge to the original home countries of the neem tree to encourage people there to not only use these valuable trees as firewood, shade, and medicine, but to also use their products as insecticides.

# Parts of Neem

## Core

The core of the neem fruit is surrounded by a skin under which there are often two or three seeds. The seeds contain a large portion of plant oil that is made up of approximately forty different ingredients. Neem oil can be extracted from the seeds by pressing or by extraction with hexane, an organic solvent.

Pressing of the neem seeds is the less aggressive procedure and produces a more valuable oil. The hexane extraction delivers higher yields; however, the oil maintains more residue and is of a noticeably inferior quality. This oil should be used only for industrial applications.

At room temperature, neem oil is solid and has the viscosity of margarine. At about twenty-three degrees Celsius, the oil melts and forms a yellowish or brown fluid with a green tint. Neem oil has a scent somewhere between that of peanuts and garlic. This scent is not to everyone's liking, but it can be removed by the addition of alcohol.

The active ingredients of neem seeds are soluble in water;

however, they are more easily soluble in alcohol or other natural solvents. For the farmer or gardener, the water solution is recommended since anyone can produce it without too much effort. For industrial usage, however, other solutions are better since they stabilize the active ingredients and facilitate the storage of ingredients.

Before the neem seeds are processed, the fruit has to be separated from the core. This is primarily done through rubbing or washing. While this sounds simple, it is quite complicated: the seeds cannot simply be dried in bags or buckets but have to be spread out thinly. Since the active ingredients in neem are sensitive to light, the seeds cannot be dried under the sun, but have to be spread out under a roof providing shade.

In countries such as India, this process is exceedingly complicated during the monsoon months. If the neem seeds are not completely dry, they are susceptible to fungi. This not only spoils them for use as a pesticide, but also poses a serious danger for humans since neem seeds carrying fungi contain carcinogenic substances and other poisons (including mycotoxins). In India, even small children are fed neem oil as a type of cure-all. When fungi-carrying neem seeds are used for the production of these oils, this "medicine" can cause severe liver and brain damage. Some children have died.

Neem seeds are also used for the creation of new plants. In the wild, neem seeds itself very quickly, usually within a few weeks, and loses its ability to germinate. Only under special storage conditions, in darkness and at cool temperatures, can neem seeds remain viable for several years.

## SEEDS

The most frequently used part of the neem tree is the fruits, or more specifically, the seeds. They contain a potpourri of ingredients that can be used for medical as well as cosmetic purposes. Furthermore, they are well suited to be used as an insecticide.

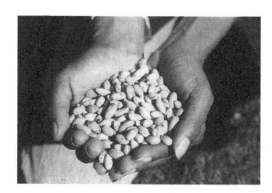

Neem seeds contain about forty active ingredients as well as a considerable amount of plant oil, which is best obtained through careful cold-pressing.

Most active ingredients in neem chemically belong to two molecular groups, the triterpenes and limonoids. Triterpenes are natural substances that often carry out the same functions as hormones. Limonoids are molecular relatives of the monoterpene limones that can be found in many essential oils and are used to test for termites. The strongest effects are believed to come from four neem ingredients: azadirachtin, meliantriol, salannin, and nimbin (or nimbidin). The effects against harmful insects are especially attributed to azadirachtin.

Neem fruits are generally harvested when they exhibit the typical yellow-green color. Since flowers and fruits can occur simultaneously on a tree, on many neem plantations there is no fixed harvesttime; rather, fruits are collected throughout the year. The fruits are often painstakingly harvested by hand. Another method consists of strongly shaking trees or branches with ripe fruits. The fruits can then be picked up from the ground. If this method is used the fruits should be picked up right away since the seeds may have already started to grow fungi.

Only when the seeds have been thoroughly dried can they be placed into bags or other containers. Seeds obtained by these means remain effective for at least two years, making storage of the seeds possible. Long and time-intensive transportation are no problem for dried neem seeds, either. They can, for example, be transported by ship from South America, saving natural resources; they do not need to be flown in by airplane.

While in principle the active ingredients could be obtained from the whole seed, the yield would be much lower, similar to making coffee with whole, unground beans. Before you pass up the use of neem completely, you are better off using whole or pressed neem seeds that have been opened by some mechanical means—for example, by having been stepped on.

Neem seeds are relatively easily ground by hand using rather basic mills. Usually the seeds are thrown into a funnel, at the end of which is a sharp-bladed screw. Turning this screw breaks up the seeds. The pieces then fall into the container.

For private use it is, of course, possible to grind neem seeds using a coffee grinder. It is, however, advisable to clean the grinder carefully afterward, since the neem otherwise causes a bitter aftertaste. While neem residues are not harmful, they can thoroughly dampen the enjoyment of a good cup of coffee. On an industrial scale, primarily electric mills are used.

## GROUND SEEDS

Ground neem seeds, just like the whole ones, have to be protected from direct sunlight and wetness, since UV rays and water accelerate the deterioration of active neem ingredients. To retain their effectiveness for as long as possible, neem products should be carefully guarded against sunlight and stored in a dry place.

Since humidity damages neem flour, the liquid solutions prepared with ground seeds are only effective for a limited period of time. Without additional stabilization, their effectiveness is quickly lost since even when they are stored cool and dry, the solution will last only about one to two weeks.

Neem seeds should not be ground too fine since this makes it harder to separate solid seed components from water later on.

Pollen-sized particles are ideal for easily filtering out with a cloth, fine gauze, a tea sieve, or even a pair of nylons. Remaining seed particles should not be thrown away since they can be used for systemic ground treatment.

## OIL

Everywhere the neem tree grows people use its seeds to obtain oil. The oil content of its seeds is around 40 to 50 percent, which makes the neem tree an important provider of oil. Aside from the technical application, neem oil also plays an important role in plant protection.

The neem seeds selected for oil production are stored for three to six months after the harvest—until they are thoroughly dry and ready for processing. The quantity of oil produced in different countries varies considerably. In Africa, neem oil is produced mostly to cover the demand of the landowner. In India and in the Caribbean, neem oil is an important export.

In poor agricultural enterprises, the processing of oil is still painstaking manual labor. First, the hard seed shells have to be removed because they make the pressing harder and lower the yield. Then, the seeds are broken up in simple hand-powered mills or even by hand with a mortar and pestle. After repeated sieving of the shells, one finally obtains the pure seeds.

The seeds are then ground thoroughly and mixed with water. Adding water makes the work easier since the neem oil melts at twenty-three degrees Celsius. The water allows the neem porridge to turn into a malleable paste that is much more easily pressed.

Wood presses operated manually or powered by oxen are widely used. The yield can be up to 100 millimeters for one kilogram of seeds. The oil rests for a few days and is then filtered.

Higher yields can be obtained using machine-powered corn mills for the cracking and sorting of the seeds, but because of expense, their usage is not profitable for a small enterprise. The formation of cooperatives would allow such use.

The temperatures used during the pressing have a strong effect on the quality of the oil obtained. At temperatures of up to seventy degrees Celsius, the oil is still considered to have been cold pressed. The incentive for the use of higher temperatures lies in the higher yield. The oil quality deteriorates at temperatures over 100 degrees Celsius, and its effectiveness suffers because of the destruction of biologically active components. When buying neem oil, you should always read the manufacturing information.

The traditional as well as the mechanized cold-pressing process delivers a high-quality oil. It has a dark yellow color, turns solid at temperatures below twenty-three degrees Celsius, and does not dry out. The oil is composed mainly of glycerides of palmitin, stearin, oil, and linol acids. It chemically resembles soy oil or olive oil. In the cold-pressed oil, there are also 10 to 20 percent of the total content of biologically active components, especially the limonoids. The rest remains in the residue.

One alternative to oil production by pressing is the extraction of the seeds with hexane. This procedure yields an oil of lower quality that can be used for mechanical purposes. Higher grade oil can be obtained through a two-step extraction: first the scent and bitter materials are extracted from the seeds with the use of alcohol, and afterward the oil is extracted with hexane. Even though this method yields good oil, only small amounts are produced by these means since the necessary solutions are expensive, and the required technical facilities are often not available.

Bitter components contained in neem oil and certain sulfur compounds that give the oil its strong garlic scent, destroy the taste. For this reason, in its raw state, neem is not used as food but is only used as grease, for wax production, as fuel (for example, for oil lamps), and in soap production. In India household soaps are produced almost exclusively with neem and coconut oil since the two substances are readily available, cheap to produce, and very effective as soap.

Because of its antiseptic qualities, neem oil is also well suited for medicinal soaps and pharmaceuticals such as salves and creams. Neem oil is used in cosmetics for creams, lotions, and shampoos. However, for these purposes, the oil is further prepared, for example, by means of distillation. This yields a finer, odorless oil with a longer shelf life since the acids responsible for its decay are also removed when the oil is distilled. The unpleasant odor of neem oil can also be eliminated by means of alcohol.

## Oil Manufacturing By-products

The dark brown residue that is left over in the production of neem oil has many uses. On a large industrial scale, the oil remaining in the residue is extracted with hexane. The oil, however, is of low quality and only suited for soaps and mechanical uses.

The neem residue also has valuable uses as a fertilizer: it contains more nitrogen, phosphorus, calcium, and magnesium than agricultural fertilizer or sludge from sewage treatment plants. There are also many valuable limonoids. Because of these ingredients, the neem residue, worked into the ground, successfully kills living nematodes such as termites at the roots of plants.

The neem residue also amplifies the fertilizing characteristics of regular urine fertilizer. This is because bacteria living in the ground process a part of the bound nitrogen contained in urine fertilizer into gaseous nitrogen. This escapes into the atmosphere or remains as a useless gas in the ground. The ingredients of the residue slow the activity of the bacteria and thus amplify the characteristics of the urine fertilizer.

Neem residue is often available in ground-up form in stores. Experts are currently testing the use of its active ingredients isolated with the use of acetone or ethanol. Their goal is the lowering of transportation costs since it would no longer be necessary to transport the entire residue but merely the extracted concentrate, which nevertheless has to be produced with expensive solvents.

## LEAVES

Even though neem leaves mixed with stored wheat and legumes have for a long time served as protection against storage parasites in India, their qualities as insecticides received no attention until about fifteen years ago. Up to then, it was mainly neem seeds that were used for plant protection and to fight vermin. Despite the fact that neem leaves do not contain exactly the same active ingredients as the seeds, they can have similar, if weaker, effects in many of the same areas. This conclusion is what the first research at the Venezuelan neem project (see case study) indicates.

Biologist Veronica Seher from Caracas is partly responsible for this. Even though the main ingredient of the neem seeds, the azadirachtin, is not found in the leaves, the biologist reports that the leaves nonetheless exhibit similar effects. Various chemical connections between the limonoids and triterpenes in the leaves are probably the cause of these comparable reactions. The harvest of the leaves of the neem trees, however, leads to lower seed yields. For this reason, the use of neem leaves has so far not been widely propagated.

In contrast to the seeds, the leaves have a pleasant odor that is important for their application in cosmetics. The extract from the neem leaves can be prepared as a tea as well as an alcoholic tincture. The alcohol extract has a dark green color and can be stored for several weeks. Water-based neem leaf extract, on the other hand, has to be further processed quickly since it retains its effectiveness for only a few weeks. Cold leaf extracts quickly ferment and are therefore not recommended.

Neem leaf extracts also demonstrate a surprising effect on the fungus *Aspergillus flavus*, which quickly spreads on our foodstuffs: the extracts keep it from producing the highly toxic aflatoxin and thereby render the fungus harmless. Aflatoxin is considered one of the most dangerous carcinogens.

In spite of their fungicidal effects, the leaves and the seeds can also fall prey to this fungus if they are not carefully dried and stored.

## BARK

The neem tree has a hard and somewhat thick brown bark. It is marked by many lines. Much like the leaves and seeds, it contains special active ingredients. In India, neem bark and branches have traditionally been used for oral hygiene and treating gum infections because of their antiseptic qualities.

In rural areas, small neem branches often replace the toothbrush: many Indians massage their gums with branches that have been shaped into brushes. Of course the small strings clean the teeth as well as the gaps between the teeth. Even though oral hygiene there does not include toothbrush and toothpaste, people generally have healthy teeth and gums.

Neem has also been processed into toothpaste. The effective ingredients are concentrated mainly in the bast (the strong fiber) of the bark, in its outermost layer. Therefore, people in India who no longer reach for neem branches need not miss its powerful effects. It's no wonder that in India toothpaste containing neem became an instant success. However, this toothpaste tastes of garlic and is slightly bitter since the bark, like the wood, the leaves, and the seeds, contains strong, pungent odors.

The first neem toothpastes are now also available on the German and U.S. markets. With essential oils and other additives, these products have a pleasant taste. Scientific studies attest to their protective effects against cavities and gum infections and also attribute a healing effect to the toothpaste.

## A VERSATILE WOOD

Neem trees provide excellent building material. The trunks are straight and have almost no knots in the lower area. Neem wood can also be manufactured into furniture. Because many pest control characteristics are inherent in the wood, it resists termites and wood worms. Fast-growing neem can be harvested after five to seven years for wood production.

However, the valuable wood by no means always ends up as building material. It is often used as firewood. For many people at the border of the Sahara, the lack of firewood is an ongoing problem. The vegetation in these latitudes is often permanently damaged by the collection of firewood. The neem tree can serve as a rotating wood provider: cut neem trees are quickly replaced by new ones. For example, it was possible to obtain 169 square meters of wood per hectare in Nigeria and 120 in Ghana within just a few years.

Nevertheless, complete clear-cutting should be avoided even with the neem tree. Because neem seeds are sensitive to light, they quickly lose their ability to germinate on the bare ground, so a neem forest will not develop in a clear-cut area. In this case, concentrated reforestation and watering would be necessary.

# CASE STUDY: ECOLOGY AND ECONOMY

A few years ago, I visited a neem project of the Friedrich-Naumann Foundation in northern Venezuela, in the community of Dabajuro. At the time of my visit, the project had only been in place for four years but showed remarkable results. Even though the north of Venezuela has always been a very hot area, in the recent past agriculture once again become possible. A short review of the history of Venezuela shows how this came about.

## PETROLEUM—A SHORT-LIVED BLESSING

In the 1970s Venezuela experienced an oil boom as petroleum was extracted in large quantities. The population left their fields and moved to the large cities since work in oil refineries and fields provided better pay than traditional agriculture. Large cities such as Caracas that were already home to millions quickly became metropolises. During this time, life in Venezuela shifted from being largely rural to being predominantly urban.

Mismanagement and confusing politics first brought about the country's exclusion from OPEC (Organization of Petroleum Exporting Countries). After this, Venezuela was unable to join

After only four years, the neem project of the cooperative El Buchal in Venezuela was successful: the neem tree made it possible to use soil damaged by erosion once again for agricultural purposes.

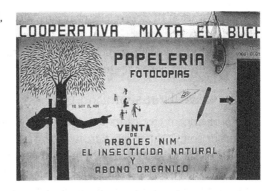

any other organization of petroleum-producing countries, and oil prices started to tumble. At the same time, its oil reserves became depleted. While Venezuela still produces a significant amount of oil, the output has fallen to a fraction of its initial production.

The people who had believed in oil for the most part lost their jobs. This is why many of them live in the Bareras, the slums, that have developed around large cities like Caracas. Thefts and robberies are a part of daily life there since the inhabitants are unable to guarantee their survival by other means. The people cannot return to the countryside since the idle fields are by now completely dried up and washed out.

Even though there is rain in some areas of Venezuela, for example in the Falcon state in the north, the ground is unable to absorb the water. Hydrology professor Saulo Olavarrieta of the university in Barquisimeto researched this phenomenon and found out that due to the lack of vegetation, there is a freshwater shortage.

Along the coast, the annual rainfall is only around 200 to 250 millimeters. While annual rainfall along the mountain regions is around 900 millimeters, this only occurs in particular areas in the form of torrential rainfalls. The water does not soak into the arid soil, but rather flows off the surface from the higher lying areas to the sea and is thus lost.

In addition, the ground is in danger of becoming too salty:

the exploitation of deep wells near agricultural fields has lowered the level of the groundwater. In some areas, sea water has already flowed in, which, because of its high concentration of salt, renders the ground infertile.

## SAVIOR IN TIMES OF NEED

While the neem tree cannot do anything about the increasing salt in the soil, it can at least grow on the extremely dry ground already damaged by erosion. This is the starting point of the project of the Friedrich-Naumann Foundation, begun eight years ago, that takes place in cooperation with the El Buchal cooperative in Dabajuro.

If you visit the Finca, the farm, today, you will find about eleven thousand neem trees. Guests are welcome as the participants of the project are proud of their work and have every reason to be: the trees are growing well; the seeds and leaves are already being processed.

When I first visited the Finca, I was surprised: individual neem trees carry names. In front of each tree was a sign, and some of the names were very familiar to me. Politicians, employees of the Friedrich-Naumann Foundation, and neem researchers have planted trees—including Professor Heinrich Schmutterer of the University Giessen. Probably the most important neem researcher, Schmutterer has devoted most of his professional life to the research of the neem tree.

I am now included in this prominent circle. I discovered a hole in the ground, and a worker from the cooperative placed a young neem tree in my hand.

The project on the Finca started in 1992 with the planting of six thousand trees. The original idea was to provide shade and to stop the erosion so that at some point in time agriculture could once again take place beneath these trees. The trees already produce so many fruits and seeds that insecticides can be extracted from them. On the Finca, seeds are dried, ground in a hand-powered mill similar to an oversized meat grinder, and then mixed with water.

Visitors on the Finca, like Ellen Norten, are always welcome. They can participate in the success of the cooperative by planting their own neem tree.

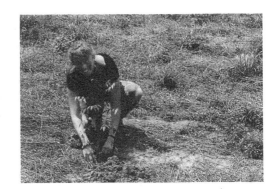

Dr. Bastian Kaiser, a participant in the neem project, is an established forest ranger. To him, the quality and appearance of the wood are, of course, of special interest, but even under his critical eyes, the neem tree gains approval. The light wood reminds most observers of maple; it is very hard and especially well suited for furniture.

When the Venezuelan trees were one year old, they stood three to four meters high. The rate of growth of the trees depends on the quality of the soil. Dr. Kaiser is researching which conditions are best suited for rapid growth of trees aimed at wood production. Individual trees are marked according to various criteria and selected for continued growth.

Dr. Kaiser and his colleagues want to find out whether the genes of these future generations will determine if the tree will grow straight and largely free of branches. Some trees give the impression that in five or six years their trunks will grow to be five or six meters high without any branches.

In an extremely dry climate and on sandy ground, even the neem tree has to be watered at first. However, a straightforward spraying is sufficient. With a simple system, the water is pumped through hoses from a nearby lake. The pump is powered by a windmill made out of cut-up oil barrels that catch the wind.

In the first four years, the initial six thousand neem trees grew to eleven thousand. But not all of the trees were planted.

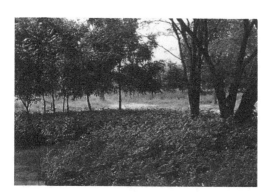

Within the first four years, the initial 6,000 trees increased to 11,000. Birds helped. They eat only the flesh of the fruit and spread the seeds on the ground.

Birds that have come to the Finca unintentionally help with the spread of the neem trees: they eat the fruits of the neem and drop the seeds on the ground, where they then start to grow. Wild neem trees, those that were "planted" by birds, can be recognized because they do not stand neatly in rows but grow randomly around the farm.

Aside from birds there are, of course, other animals that enjoy life on the Finca. Every once in a while, the head of an iguana can be seen popping out from among the leaves of a tree. Only one animal is missed here at first glance: goats. While there are goats milling about almost everywhere in the region—their number is estimated at several million—these hungry animals do not roam here. Only after prolonged searching do you find these indispensable, useful animals on the Finca.

Usually people in northern Venezuela build fences around their houses to protect themselves against the free-running goats since they eat the ground bare. People who want to have even a single flower in front of their house need to build fences. In the project this situation is reversed: the fence does not keep the goats out, but in. The animals cannot move about freely anymore and are thereby kept from causing damage. On the Finca, which spans almost ninety hectares, the goats still have enough space in their enclosures to find all the food they need.

The enclosure of these animals also provides an opportunity

The important but gluttonous goats of the cooperative are kept in large enclosures to protect the neem trees from their voracious appetites.

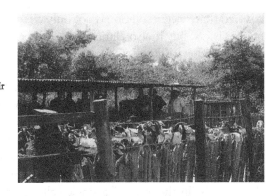

to learn more about their nutritional needs. The health of the goats is also more easily managed. The success of the enclosure for the neem project is indisputable: surely many of the neem trees would no longer have such thick foliage if the goats were free to roam about.

## Neem for Goats

Fleas, lice, and ticks among goats can easily be treated using neem. This is possible with a watery neem solution, but Veronica Seher, a cosmetic specialist and natural healer in the neem project in Venezuela, developed an even more effective neem shampoo based on the results of her research. Goats and, of course, other animals that are victim to the ectoparasites have already been treated successfully. This success is also an economic success: here in the hot areas in Falcon goat keeping is especially threatened by skin parasites. Neem shampoo provides a welcome solution for the entire region.

The goats benefit from the neem trees in two regards. While the neem project does not finance any related research, in 1993, three veterinarians joined the cooperative to collect data for their dissertations. Neem seeds were made available to the young scientists in order for them to perform their own related experiments in the project.

During the course of these experiments, the scientists discovered that a neem solution is not only effective against external parasites, but it also eliminates a number of internal parasites, or endoparasites.

Hygiene and sanitary facilities for animals on Falcon have traditionally been criminally neglected. The most important animals, goats and cattle, are severely affected by parasitic organisms and especially worms. Their metabolism is disrupted as a result, and they cannot make use of all nutrients even when fed well. The fur of the animals then loses its shine and starts to shed.

The majority of parasites can be found in the intestines of the animals. In the feces of a single calf, up to sixteen million worm eggs were found by the young researchers. Such a strong parasitic influence can often lead to the death of the animal. When they discovered this, the young scientists were moving into new territory. The effects of the watered down neem extracts on internal parasites had up to then hardly been researched. They proved the effectiveness of the neem solution; they now have to find the right dosage for a worm treatment.

One of the young scientists is Miguel Delmoral of the university in Coro. He reported, "We first used a minimal dosage on the animals, but we were disappointed to observe that with these small doses the number of parasites actually increased. We were about to abandon our studies in this area. But instead we increased the dosage in a series of small steps and reached a point where our cure shows solid success."

The experiments showed that the nematode incidents had been lowered significantly through the usage of neem. Goats reacted to this treatment noticeably better than cattle even though both animals had the same type of nematode. "What neem ingredients cause these changes will be explored in further studies," Miguel Delmoral enthusiastically explained.

"In any case, we have to continue our research because we worked completely independently, without any additional scientific support from our university in Coro," he continued. "We also finished the first part of our study in the summertime. Thus we do not know in what form the climate of this dry period influenced our results. We have to continue our study in what is called winter here, in the rainy season, and then compare our results with those of the summer."

## PLAY IN THE SHADE OF NEEM TREES

Enthusiasm for the neem tree is by no means held solely by scientists or by people closely involved in this project; it has long since spread past the Finca. Dabajuro, the town in the desert, is once again green. Neem trees can be found everywhere: cab drivers park their cars in the shade of a neem and wait on a bench for the next fare. The Plaza Bolivar, the central meeting point in town, has been greened by the trees, and even in front of individual residences, the trees are growing to remarkable sizes.

The cooperative El Buchal played a part in this: neem trees are planted in all residential areas where the neem idea was welcome. There are no costs involved for the people living in these neighborhoods since the cooperative donates the trees.

Each inhabitant in Dabajuro can thus enjoy the benefits of the neem project. The driving theory behind the project is this: Once one has seen the advantages of the neem tree, one is more likely to protect the environment and become an advocate of neem trees. Children too are getting to know and love the neem tree. Colored pictures on walls of plants and neem trees serve as educational material and provide fun and games in the kindergarten.

Teacher Nelida Cuenca de Reyes, who the children lovingly call Nelly, reported the reactions of the students to the neem trees in the garden: "They are very happy to play in the shade under trees. We often see that they even eat the fruits, that they are able to quickly separate the fruit from the core. And the little ones, the five-year olds, the older ones, by now know that the neem trees offer various possibilities for applications—medical healing ones and others. They themselves have already planted trees as well, and we have helped them with it." Five-year-old Orlando proudly presented me,

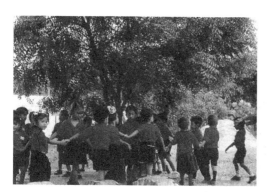

Not only scientists are enthusiastic about the neem tree. People everywhere in Dabajuro enjoy the refreshing shade of the fast-growing trees.

the visitor, with "his" tree behind the kindergarten building.

The neem trees also specifically help to support the kindergarten. Money is scarce; with the neem seeds and the sale of young trees, at least a modest amount of money can be earned.

Enthusiastically, Nelly continued to report: "It really is an important source of funds for us. We are on our own here and planting these trees not only provides us with shade, we can also use the seeds for different applications. As teachers, we pass on the knowledge about neem and teach the community what the neem tree is useful for. And we have a source of funds, we can sell them, and we can plant our gardens and our community with trees."

The idea of neem seems to have infected most people in this city in Venezuela. And for some, the work in the cooperative has also helped in overcoming personal problems. For a long time former policeman Clemente Artenga had difficult problems in his family. During this hard time, the work on the neem project gave him something to hold on to. Many participants in the project were motivated by the commitment of the coordinator. To his colleagues, Clemente Artenga has long been "Commandante Nim." He enjoys the nickname.

## PROOF OF SUCCESS

The first successes of the project fill the volunteer participants of the cooperative with pride. Many Venezuelans first frowned upon

"Commandante Nim" is one of the many people that contribute to the success of the cooperative El Buchal.

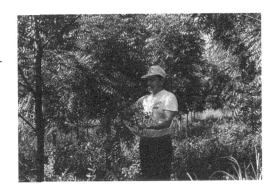

the cooperative; they even looked down upon the activity. "Trees won't grow in the desert" said the skeptics. Today the proof is everywhere: the yields from the neem plantation are so great that the export of neem seed to the international market is in the works.

The neem project in Dabajuro is only one of many neem projects around the globe. Often neem projects are part of development aid because the neem tree in many areas allows people one avenue to self-sufficiency. Gerhard Schnepel of the Friedrich-Naumann Foundation is cofounder of the project. As a veteran in the area of development aid politics, he explained that "it is of great importance that economical activities take place in context with ecological concerns. There has to be a connection between ecology and economy. The neem tree is especially well suited for this." Schnepel emphasized in our discussion that "the tree is not only ecologically extremely interesting as a source of natural insecticides, but also has an economical perspective since the marketing of neem trees from the plantations in the project allow for revenue essential to raise the standard of living in those places."

It is likely that people in other neem projects are just as enthusiastic as the people in Dabajuro. In the Dominican Republic, Costa Rica, Honduras, and Nicaragua, as well as in a number of African countries, neem projects are under way, many of which have already expanded into successful enterprises.

# MEDICINAL USES OF NEEM

3

Neem, known as the Village Pharmacy, has long been used in both traditional and modern medicine. In Sanskrit, neem is known as *sarva roga nivarini,* "the curer of all ailments." The first indication that it was being used medicinally was about 4,500 years ago, in India. Excavations at Harappa and at Mohenjo-Daro, in the northwestern and western parts of the country, uncovered several therapeutic compounds, some of which included neem leaves. Early Indian Vedic medical practitioners moved directly to clinical trials rather than to laboratory studies. The tests took dozens of scientists hundreds of years to finish. As there were no pharmaceutical companies and no malpractice suits, they had the time and freedom to experiment until they found the best medical solution.

In ancient documents that have been translated, such as the Caraka-Samhita, written in approximately 500 B.C., and Susruta Samhita, written in approximately A.D. 300 (they may both be much earlier), the foundation for the Indian system of natural healing, Ayurveda, is explained. Ayurveda, a five-thousand-year-old healing system, considers health as a reflection of the proper

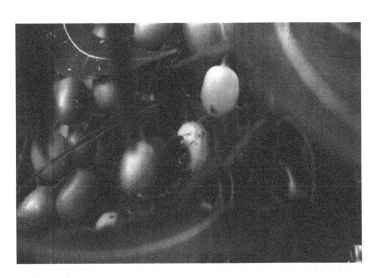

The fruits, or rather the seeds, of the neem tree contain a potpourri of active ingredients, which can be used for medicinal or cosmetic applications as well as in the protection of plants.

balance of life forces in a person. Neem is mentioned in almost one hundred entries for treating a wide variety of diseases and symptoms. During that time in history, neem provided virtually an entire health program and was a part of almost every aspect of life in many parts of India. In much of the country, it still does just that.

Here are some examples: The Sarira Sthanam recommended that newborns be anointed with herbs and oil, laid on a sheet of silk, and fanned with a leafy branch of neem. When the child fell ill, he was given small doses of neem oil. He was bathed in neem tea to treat cuts and lesions from chicken pox, and he and his parents brushed their teeth daily with neem twigs. The myriad of applications go on, until at death, neem branches covered the body, and neem wood was burned in the funeral pyre. When people return from funerals, they keep neem leaves in their mouths, signifying grief.

Almost all parts of the tree are useful in treating a variety of human health conditions. A 10 percent aqueous extract of neem's tender leaves has been found to possess antiviral properties. Neem is often used in the case of poisonous bites. Neem leaf extract contains a clotting inhibitor. An extract of neem leaves has shown potential as a powerful hepatoprotective (liver protecting) agent. The essential oil from its fresh leaves has a mild fungicidal action.

Its fruit and seeds are powerful, as well. Gedunin, present in the fruit, has been shown to possess antimalarial activity. The dry fruits are bruised in water for use in treating skin diseases. Among more than one hundred compounds found in neem are azadirachtins from the seed kernel. So far, twelve azadirachtins have been identified, all of which exhibit a high level of biological activity. The kernels produce a brown, bitter, fixed oil called Oil of Margosa. The oil possesses antifungal and antiseptic qualities and is considered to have antifertility properties.

The bark's nimibidin, known to be antipyretic and a nonirritant, has been found useful to treat skin disease, burn ulcers, herpes labialis, scabies, and more. Extracts of the bark have powerful diuretic and anti-inflammatory properties.

According to Ayurvedic sources, neem is a powerful blood purifier and detoxifier. It reduces fever and toxins involved in most inflammatory skin diseases and is effective in the treatment of malaria; its astringent action promotes healing; it is used to treat skin diseases, parasites, thirst, nausea, arthritis, rheumatism, and much more. Neem stimulates the production of T-cells to fight infections. It boosts the immune system on all levels while helping the body fight infection. Modern usages include those for various cancers and for AIDS.

Neem, however, must be used cautiously in cases of extreme fatigue or emaciation. It may become toxic if ingested in extremely large amounts. As with most substances, a person should first undertake a neem regimen in small quantities. Although side effects are extremely rare, one should evaluate one's body's reactions and continue accordingly.

A wide multitude of diseases or conditions can be successfully treated with various elements of neem.

# AIDS

Some of the best news is that neem may help in the search for a prevention or a cure for AIDS. So far, the National Institutes of Health reports encouraging results from in vitro tests for an AIDS prevention and possible cure using extracts from the tree. Professionally administered neem solutions are currently being studied for their effects on cancer, diabetes, heart disease, and AIDS. In 1993, in a preliminary study, the National Institutes of Health reported positive results from in vitro tests where neem bark extracts killed the AIDS virus. Using extracts made by soaking neem bark in water, Dr. Van Der Nat of the Netherlands found that the extract produced a strong immune stimulating reaction. Studies reported in 1992 and 1994 showed neem's ability to enhance the cell-mediated immune response may be used to provide protection from vaginal contraction of the disease if neem is used as a vaginal lubricant preceding intercourse. AIDS may possibly be treated by ingesting neem leaf extracts or the whole leaf or by drinking a neem tea.

Neem contains immune modulating polysaccharide compounds; this polysaccharide may be responsible for increasing antibody production. Other elements of neem may stimulate immune function by enhancing cellular mediated response. This dual action can help the body ward off the frequent infections that generally accompany AIDS.

## ARTHRITIS

Neem has a long history of relieving inflamed joints, supported by recent scientific studies. Most anti-inflammatories, such as aspirin and ibuprofen, irritate the stomach and may be the major cause for upper GI bleeding. Ulcers sometimes occur as a result of taking too much of these over-the-counter drugs. Neem is comparably effective to phenyl butazone or cortisone as an anti-inflammatory and does not adversely affect the stomach. The active constituents in its leaves relieve pain by acting on the prostaglandin mechanism and significantly reduce acute edema.

Several studies have shown its usefulness with this disease. Some studies have looked at the ability of neem leaf extracts to reduce inflammation. One suggested that the phenolic compounds containing catechin (which possesses anti-inflammatory properties) may produce the anti-inflammatory effects. Another investigation found that quercetin, an antibacterial compound, exists in neem's leaves. Other studies have shown that the polysaccharides in neem reduce the inflammation and swelling that occur in arthritis.

Not only does neem help reduce inflammation, it also has pain-suppressing properties. Neem can also help create a balance in the immune system, directly affecting the progression of arthritis.

## Birth Control

Neem has been shown to be a powerful, relatively inexpensive birth control agent for both men and women. In the first century B.C., Charaka, the Indian physician, gave a detailed method for using neem for contraception. Cotton soaked in neem oil was kept in the vagina for fifteen minutes before intercourse. This killed the sperm.

In both India and the United States, trials show neem extract reduces fertility in male monkeys without inhibiting libido or sperm production. Also, in other Indian studies, neem leaf tablets taken for one month produced reversible male infertility but did not affect sperm production or libido. This shows promise as the first male birth control pill.

In another study, members of the Indian Army were tested with neem's birth control effects. Twenty married men took daily oral doses of several drops of neem seed oil in gelatin capsules. To become 100 percent effective, the effect took six weeks, but it remained effective during the entire year of the trial, and was only reversed six weeks after a man no longer took the capsules. The men experienced no adverse side effects and retained their normal capabilities and desires. No women became pregnant during this period. This product is now offered in stores under the name "Sensal."

It appears that a tiny amount of neem oil injected in the vas deferens might be able to provide up to eight months of birth control. Tests in this area revealed no obstructions, no change in testosterone production, and no antisperm antibodies. The local lymph nodes showed an increased ability to respond to infections, indicating an immune response that might be responsible for the birth control effect.

Neem's contraceptive uses for women are even more varied. Even the leaves are said to be effective. Many women in Madagascar chew a handful of neem leaves every day, which, according to their statements, prevents pregnancies. In the case of unwanted pregnancies, neem is said to be capable of inducing a miscarriage.

Neem oil-based vaginal creams and suppositories are extremely popular in India. Nonirritating and easy to use, they are almost 100 percent effective. When tested against human sperm, neem extract (sodium nimbidinate) at 1,000 mg was able to kill all sperm in five minutes and required only 30 minutes at a lower, 250 mg, level. It is suggested that these creams and suppositories also prevent vaginal and sexually transmitted diseases.

Several years of study in India by leading scientists resulted in a neem-based polyherbal vaginal cream with both spermicidal and antimicrobial action. The studies proved that neem oil killed sperm in the vagina within thirty seconds and was effective up to five hours. Many other spermicide creams must be reapplied at least hourly. Neem oil, when used in the vagina, seems to increase the antigen presenting ability of the uterine tract. This apparently has a direct spermicidal effect without known side effects.

The cream contains 25 percent neem seed extract along with extracts from the soap nut and from quinine hydrochloride. Based on these experiments, a neem-based contraceptive cream was developed by an Indian pharmaceutical company. It tested to be safer and easier to use than chemical-based foams and gels, was nearly 100 percent effective, and was used more frequently than the alternatives. Its effect does not appear to be hormonal, and the product is considered a safe alternative to other methods that employ hormones.

Oddly, neem oil has also been taken internally by ascetics who wish to diminish their sexual desire.

## CANCER

Throughout Southeast Asia neem has been used successfully by herbalists for hundreds of years to reduce tumors. Researchers are now supporting these uses. Neem has been tested on many types of cancers, such as skin cancers, using neem-based creams, and lymphocytic cancer, using the herb internally. In India, Europe, and Japan, scientists have found that polysaccharides and limonoids in neem bark, leaves, and seed oil reduced tumors and cancers and were effective against lymphocytic leukemia.

In Japan, several issued patents included hot water neem bark extracts; these were effective against several types of cancer. Several extracts were tested at different doses and were compared to standard anticancer agents. Many extracts were equal or better than the standard treatments against solid tumors. Results of tests performed with a more purified extract of the bark produced even better results. Further studies using pure active compounds are hoped to produce even more impressive results.

In another study, one researcher used an extract of neem leaves to prevent the adhesion of cancer cells to other body cells. If cancers can't stick to other cells, the cancer can't spread throughout the body and is more easily destroyed.

Neem's success has been noticeably remarkable with skin

cancers. A number of reports have been made by patients that their skin cancers have disappeared after several months of using a neem-based cream on a daily basis. Injections of neem extract around various tumors have shown sizable reduction in a few weeks' time.

## Dental Care

People in both India and Africa have used neem twigs as tooth brushes for centuries. Neem twigs contain antiseptic ingredients necessary for dental hygiene. Neem powder is also used to brush teeth and massage gums.

Other countries are beginning to follow their lead. In Germany, researchers have shown that neem extracts prevent tooth decay and periodontal disease. In the United States, more than 90 percent of the adult population today have some sort of periodontal disease. Infections, tooth decay, bleeding and sore gums have all been treated successfully with daily use of neem mouth rinse or neem leaf extract added to the water. Some people have reported a total reversal of gum degeneration after using neem for only a few months.

## Diabetes

Because neem is a tonic and a revitalizer, it works effectively in the treatment of diabetes, as well. More than a disease that requires change of diet, diabetes is the leading cause of blindness in people ages twenty-five to seventy-four; it also damages nerves, kidneys, the heart, and blood vessels; it may even result in the loss of limbs. Incurable, it can be treated in a variety of ways. One recommendation is to take one tablespoon (5 ml) of neem leaf juice daily on an empty stomach each morning for three months. An alternative is to chew or take in powder form ten neem leaves daily in the morning. Some studies have shown that oral application of neem leaf extracts reduced a patient's insulin requirements by between 30 and 50 percent for nonkeytonic, insulin fast, and insulin-sensitive diabetes.

Because neem has been found to reduce insulin requirements by up to 50 percent, without altering blood glucose levels, the Indian government has approved the sale of neem capsules and tablets through pharmacies and clinics for this purpose. Many of these pills are made of essentially pure, powdered neem leaves.

Karnim, one medication that contains neem and a number of other herbs, available in many countries for treating diabetes, was found to lower blood sugar by more than 50 percent in twenty weeks and to maintain that level thereafter.

## HEART DISEASE

Major causes of a heart attack include blood clots, high cholesterol, arrhythmic heart action, and high blood pressure. Neem has been helpful in these conditions, too. Its leaf extracts have reduced clotting, lowered blood pressure and bad cholesterol, slowed rapid or abnormally high heartbeat, and inhibited irregular heart rhythms. Some compounds may produce effects similar to mild sedatives, which reduce anxiety and other emotional or physical states that may prompt a heart attack. The antihistamine effects of the nimbidin in its leaves cause blood vessels to dilate. This may be why the leaves help reduce blood pressure.

A recent study proved that, when a patient took either neem leaf extract or neem capsules for a month, her high cholesterol levels fell substantially. In another study, alcoholic extract of neem leaves reduced serum cholesterol by approximately 30 percent two hours after its administration. The cholesterol level stayed low for an additional four hours until testing ceased.

Another study showed that an intravenous alcoholic extract of the leaf produced a large, immediate decrease in blood pressure, lasting for several hours. A neem leaf extract, sodium nimbidinate, given to those with congestive cardiac failure, was successful as a diuretic. Regarding arrhythmic heart action, neem leaf extract exhibited antiarrhythmic activity, which returned to normal within eight minutes of administration.

# MALARIA

According to the Neem Association, an international nonprofit organization, malaria affects hundreds of millions of people worldwide and kills more than two million every year. Because of the introduction of new mosquito strains and because of more frequent travelers from malarial regions, people in North America also now acquire this disease. Malaria is quite common in India and throughout the tropics. The disease is transmitted from an infected person to a noninfected one by the bites of a certain species of mosquito, anopheles, which live in most tropical and subtropical countries. They bite from dusk to dawn. The malarial gamete is sucked by the mosquito from the infected person and carried in the insect's gut until it bites an uninfected person. The bite injects the gamete into the blood stream; it then travels to the kidney to mature. Symptoms can develop as soon as six to eight days after being bitten by an infected mosquito or as late as several months later. It should be treated as early as possible.

Neem has been shown to be effective in a number of ways against this deadly disease. Both water and alcohol-based neem leaf extracts have been confirmed as effective. It has been shown to block the development of the gamete in an infected person.

Neem leaf extract greatly increases the state of oxidation in red blood cells, which prevents normal development of the malaria virus. Irodin A, an active ingredient in the leaves, is toxic to resistant strains of malaria; 100 percent of the malaria gamete are dead within seventy-two hours with a 1 to 20,000 ratio of active ingredients. Other experiments have used alcoholic extracts of neem leaf, which performed almost as well.

Gedunin and quercetin, compounds found in the leaves, are also effective against malaria. Several studies show that neem extracts are effective even against the more virulent strains of the malaria parasite. Some scientists believe that stimulation of the immune system is a major factor in neem's effectiveness against malaria. The plant also lowers the fever and increases one's appetite, enabling a stronger body to fight the parasite and recover more quickly.

Some westerners already familiar with neem's qualities substitute an occasional neem leaf tea for a drink of quinine when traveling to malaria-infested areas of Africa and India.

Even though neem may be effective against the parasites that carry malaria, it has not been shown to prevent the malaria infection once it's in the body.

## RHEUMATISM

Neem's leaves have anti-inflammatory activity, similar to that in drugs such as phenyl butazone and cortisone. They can relieve pain and reduce acute pain edema. For rheumatism, topical applications of a warmed neem cream that contains neem oil—and perhaps a mild neem tea—will help lessen pain. Some researchers have also indicated that a mild neem tea once a day for two weeks also helps lessen infections. After the first two weeks, you may drink the tea only every other day for two more weeks. (See our advice regarding tea on page 57.)

## STRESS

Relatively new scientific findings indicate that neem may even be useful for reducing anxiety and stress. An experiment was done on test animals to see what, if any effect neem leaf extract had on these conditions. Fresh neem leaves were crushed and the liquid squeezed out to produce a leaf extract. The extract was given orally to three main sets of animals, in two standard stress tests.

One group received salt water as a base control; another received Valium; another received the neem leaf extract. The third group was subdivided into sets that received ever larger doses. In the elevated plus maze test, doses of neem leaf extract up to 200 mg/kg showed important antianxiety activity equal to or greater than Valium. The test doses of neem leaf extract up to 100 mg/kg were equal to Valium in their antianxiety effect. At 800 mg/kg, the effects of the neem totally disappeared. Neem extracts apparently only work in small doses for this application.

The explanation of neem's antianxiety effect may be its ability to increase the amount of serotonin in the brain. Because it works well in small amounts, it could be safer than drugs currently used for stress, which may cause many side effects.

## ULCERS

In the Ayurvedic medical tradition, neem is considered a useful therapy for ulcers and gastric discomfort. Compounds in neem have been proven to have antiulcerative effects. Throughout India, people take neem leaves for all sorts of stomach problems. Some scientific evidence exists for its effectiveness for these problems. Peptic ulcers and duodenal ulcers are treated well with neem leaf extracts; nimbidin from seed extracts taken orally prevents duodenal lesions and peptic ulcers, and provides significant reductions in acid output and gastric fluid activity. Low doses of 20 to 40 mg/kg bring the most relief; increased dosages reduce the effectiveness of neem's antiulcerative effects.

Neem is also useful for treating other problems in the stomach and bowels. The herb promotes a healthy digestive system by protecting the stomach, aiding in elimination, and removing toxins and noxious bacteria. Its leaves are often used to treat heartburn and indigestion. Some neem extracts reduce the concentration of hydrochloric acid in the stomach. At the first signs of indigestion, traditional Ayurvedic practice recommends drinking a strong neem tea made of five neem leaves mixed with one-quarter teaspoon each of ginger and baking soda. This beverage supposedly protects the stomach and relieves discomfort. (See the cautions regarding neem tea on page 57.)

Neem extracts are also used to treat gastritis. The extracts reduce the amount of acid in the stomach; their antibacterial and anti-inflammatory properties can relieve the effects of this condition.

Finally, neem has also been shown to be effective for treating digestive disorders such as diarrhea, dysentery, hyperacidity, and constipation. For diarrhea and dysentery, one solution is to take one tablespoon of neem leaf juice with sugar three times a day. For constipation, a neem powder of two to three grams. with three to four black peppers given three times a day is both a laxative and a demulcent.

## VITILIGO

Vitiligo is believed to be an autoimmune disorder that causes patches of skin to lose their color. It occurs in about five percent of the human population regardless of race, but most commonly in dark-skinned people. The two most common treatments are exposure to sunlight (or PUVA) or corticosteroid drugs, but these are not always effective.

Oral doses of neem were tested at least one year on fifteen patients who had the disease. They also applied a cream made up of several herbs to patches, which were then exposed to the sun. After ninety days, 25 percent of the patients showed complete relief; another 60 percent showed mild to moderate relief. No adverse reactions were shown by any participants. Those who stayed on the treatment the longest showed the most improvement. The dosage was four grams of neem leaves three times a day, ideally taken before each meal. In the West, application of the cream is not practical as it is almost impossible to obtain. However, other studies showed that the internal use of neem leaves and bark were effective even without the cream. It may be possible that neem oil applied to the affected areas could aid in the reversal of the discoloration.

## MISCELLANEOUS HEALTH BENEFITS

Neem truly seems like a miraculous natural drug. Neem has been shown to provide an antiviral treatment option for smallpox, chicken pox, and warts. It is particularly useful for these conditions when applied directly to the skin. This is due in part to its ability to inhibit viruses from multiplying and spreading.

Chronic fatigue is considered to be caused by both viral and fungal infections. Neem, which can attack both, helps the body fight this debilitating syndrome.

Minor cuts, sprains, and bruises are treated with neem lotion, cream, or leaf extract applied locally. Its anti-inflammatory and antibacterial attributes are soothing to these conditions.

Hepatitis is another disease helped by neem. This often deadly disease can be transmitted through blood or by ingesting contaminated food or water. Recent studies indicate that neem extracts can block infection by the virus that causes the disease. Some studies have recommended drinking neem leaf tea after eating shellfish and after swimming in or drinking water that might be contaminated with sewage. (See the warning section on tea on page 57.)

Tests in Germany have shown that neem extracts are toxic to the herpes virus and can easily heal cold sores. Both a mild neem leaf tea and a topical cream application are recommended. Once the eruption has peaked, discontinue the tea (taken after breakfast and after dinner) and continue to apply cream until the sore has healed.

Chagas disease is a major health problem that infects some sixteen to eighteen million people, with another ninety million at risk in parts of South and Central America. It may be deadly. There is no vaccine and no safe and effective drug for its cure. The disease is caused by a parasite, *Trypanosoma cruzi*, which is spread by an insect, named the kissing bug.

Lab tests in Germany and Brazil have indicated that neem may be a solution. Neem leaf extracts have negative effects on these pernicious insects. Feeding neem—or more specifically a single dose of aradirachtin—to the bugs not only eliminates the parasites, but the azadirachtin prevents the young from molting and the adults from reproducing. Neem leaf or seed extracts may also be sprayed throughout the home where the kissing bug lives; this eliminates the parasites and prevents the bugs from laying eggs. Drinking neem tea may also be useful.

At the moment, scientists are researching the antibacterial and virus-reducing characteristics of the tree. The first studies confirm its effectiveness against selected fungi that occur, for example, on hair (trichophyton), skin, and nails (epidermophyton), or in the vagina (candida).

## SKIN DISEASES

Neem has been highly successful against harmful fungi, parasites, and viruses. Although it can destroy these, it does not kill off beneficial intestinal flora nor produce adverse side effects. Neem is toxic to several fungi that attack humans, including the causes of athlete's foot and ringworm, and candida, which causes yeast infections and thrush. In fact, neem extracts are some of the most powerful antifungal plant extracts found in the Indian pharmacopia that are used for these conditions. The compounds gedunin and nimbidol, found in the tree's leaves, control the fungi listed above. Basing their studies on the ancient tradition of using neem to purify the air surrounding sick people, two Indian researchers found that neem smoke was successful in suppressing fungal growth and germination.

One of neem's strongest advantages is its effect upon the skin in general. It has been most helpful in treating a variety of skin problems and diseases including psoriasis, eczema, and other persistent conditions.

According to a report from the National Research Council's Ad Hoc Panel of the Board on Science and Technology for International Development, neem preparations from the leaves or oils can be used as general antiseptics. Because neem contains antibacterial properties, it is highly effective in treating epidermal conditions such as acne, psoriasis, and eczema. It is also used for treating septic sores, infected burns, scrofula, indolent ulcers, and ringworm. Stubborn warts can be cleared up when a high-quality neem product is used. Unlike synthetic chemicals that often produce side effects such as rashes, allergic reactions, or redness, neem doesn't seem to create any of these results.

Early Ayurvedic practitioners believed high sugar levels in the body caused skin disease. Neem's bitter quality was considered to counteract the sweetness. Indians historically bathed in neem leaves steeped in hot water. This is still considered a common procedure for curing skin ailments or allergic reactions.

Psoriasis is successfully treated with neem oil. The oil moisturizes and protects the skin while healing the lesions, scaling, and irritations. Experiments have shown that patients with psoriasis who have taken neem leaf orally, combined with topical treatment with neem extracts and neem seed oil, achieve results at least as positive as those who use coal tar and cortisone, the more traditional treatments. Coal tar products are messy and smelly, and cortisone can thin the skin when used repeatedly. Neem has neither side effect. It can be used for extended periods of time without any side effects, is easy to apply, and is relatively inexpensive.

## VIRAL DISEASES

In India, neem is also used to treat viral diseases such as smallpox, chicken pox, and warts. Even many medical practitioners use a paste of neem leaves, rubbed directly on the infected skin, for these conditions. Experiments with smallpox, chicken pox, and fowlpox have shown that neem is quite effective for preventing if not for curing these conditions. The neem extracts absorb the viruses, preventing them from spreading to unaffected cells. Neem has also been shown to be effective against herpes virus and the viral DNA polymerase of the hepatitis B virus.

Veronika Seher, a participant in the neem project in Dabajuro, Venezuela (see Case Study), has developed recipes for treating fungi and skin infections that have successfully been used for some time by the participants of the project as well as by the population of Dabajuro. She made these recipes available to us.

We made slight changes in the raw materials used for cosmetics: we replaced the basic substances available in Venezuela (which unfortunately are relatively strong) with much milder substances. However, the effectiveness of the combinations is unaffected by these changes.

## Neem salve for skin fungi, small wounds, and swellings

(amounts for about 100 g cream)

> *8 g acetyl alcohol*
> *4 g neem oil*
> *4 g avocado or almond oil*
> *50 g distilled water*
> *5 g neem seeds (finely ground)*
> *5 g neem leaves (finely ground)*
> *8 g glycerin*
> *3 g zetesol*
> *5 ml xanthan*
> *10 drops palmarosa oil (Cymbopogon martinii)*
> *1 pinch natural vitamin E*

Mix the acetyl alcohol with the neem oil and avocado (or almond) oil in a water bath. In a second container, mix the water with neem seeds, and the neem leaf flour, add glycerin and zetesol and warm the mixture while stirring. Afterward add the xanthan, and stir the mixture until it thickens. Add the melted oil to this mixture, and thoroughly mix it in. Once the salve has cooled down, add the palmarosa oil and the vitamin E.

Since the seeds, leaves, and oil are combined in this cream, all of neem's active ingredients are present. That is why the cream is effective for a broad range of ailments. Its effectiveness is complemented by the palmarosa oil, which acts against viruses and also imparts a pleasant scent that drowns out most of the typical neem odor. Xanthan ensures the creamy consistency of this water-in-oil emulsion. Vitamin E preserves the mixture.

The following recipe against nail fungi also comes from Veronika Seher. Unfortunately, the basic substances in this nail polish cannot be exchanged for milder ingredients since polish can only be thinned with organic solvents. With the choice of nail polish remover or acetone, there is thus a "lazy" compromise: they belong to the less harmful organic solvents, but by no means promote health. Therefore, you should only prepare this neem solution outdoors and always cover the containers after use. Be careful not to inhale any fumes. In spite of these restrictions, neem nail polish is an effective product against resistant nail fungi for hands and feet.

### Neem nail polish for nail fungi

*15 g neem leaves (crushed)*
*5 g neem seeds (ground)*
*100 ml nail polish remover (or acetone)*
*1 bottle nail polish*

Mix the crushed neem leaves and the neem seeds with the nail polish remover, cover them, and let them sit for a day. Afterward filter them with filter paper and mix with the nail polish.

Clean your finger nails before the treatment and roughen them up a little with an emery board (use a new piece for each nail). Afterward, apply the nail polish several times. Use the nail polish until the fungi are gone.

Laboratory experiments have shown that neem has antibacterial characteristics as well. For example the bacterium *Staphylococcus aureus*, a feared cause of food poisonings as well as of furuncles and abscesses, reacted to neem treatment. Also, German experiments proved that a neem seed extract with ethanol is effective against the herpes viruses. As previously noted, Veronika Seher developed neem's disinfecting and skin care characteristics. Here is a recipe for a household and shower soap:

## Neem soap

*1 bar soap (foamy shower soap)*
*100 g neem leaf tincture*
*50 ml Face-Tensid*
*10 g (1 tablespoon) salt*
*10 ml neem oil*
*5 g perfume oil of your choice (for example, rose oil, palmarosa oil, orange oil, cedar oil)*

Chop the soap finely and melt it, together with the neem leaf tincture, in a pot while stirring constantly. Add the Face-Tensid and the salt, stir, and let cool. Once the mass is no longer hot (about forty degrees Celsius), add the neem oil and the perfume oil. Now knead the soap into a ball or pour it into a mold and let it cool.

## NEEM FOR PAIN

Because neem ingredients have a positive influence on muscle problems, Veronika Seher took this neem quality as the basis for her pressure bandage recipe. In combination with hibiscus petals, the pressure bandage is also effective against headaches.

### Neem pressure bandage for muscle pains and headaches

*200 ml boiling water*
*10 g neem leaves*
*10 g hibiscus petals*

Pour boiling water over the neem leaves and the hibiscus petals and let them sit for thirty minutes. Pour the mixture through a kitchen sieve and dip a small towel into the liquid until it is fully soaked. For pressure bandages to be applied on muscles, a warm or even hot bandage is recommended. For neck and forehead ban-

dages, a cold temperature is preferable. You can cool
the solution in the refrigerator.

## PROTECTION AGAINST PARASITES

Today, scientists are successfully testing neem oil to combat
parasites and diseases affecting plants in greenhouses and in the
outdoors. The repeated use of the oil demonstrates its effectiveness against serious plant diseases such as rust and mildew. Furthermore, the spraying of healthy plants with neem oil has served
to protect them from diseases.

Which ingredients in the oil are responsible for its protective and healing effects is unknown at this point. Therefore be
cautious: plants are very sensitive to oils, and neem oil is no
exception. The oil content of the sprayings should not exceed 2
percent. Otherwise, the oil will clog up the pores of the leaves,
the plant can no longer breathe, and it will suffocate. The alkaline effects of neem oil can also damage the plant tissue. The
applications should take place at dusk and not in the high sun
since dusk is less taxing for the plant.

Neem ingredients have been used against parasites for a long
time. Aside from an internal application, they can also be applied externally. Of course this application is by no means limited to animals; humans can also profit from neem's effects on
so-called ectoparasites.

Lice, fleas, and scabies mites are by no means a thing of
the past. In schools, these parasites can develop into serious
plagues. In a large-scale experiment in Chile in 1995, it was
possible to keep a kindergarten, otherwise frequently invaded
by parasites, completely free of these insects. As part of the
project, the children washed their hair with neem shampoo
on a regular basis.

### Neem shampoo against pests

> *10 g neem leaves (well crushed)*
> *100 ml lukewarm water*

*70 ml Face-Tensid*
*5 ml fragrance-free conditioner*
*10 g Rewoderm HT (for consistency)*
*10 drops tea tree oil*
*5 drops lemon oil*

Mix the crushed neem leaves with the water and let stand for three hours while stirring frequently. Pour through a sieve. Mix the Face-Tensid with the conditioner, which has an antielectric effect. Add the neem solution.

In order for the shampoo to be easily applied, add about ten grams of Rewoderm to the mixture. Next, add only the essential oils: 10 drops of tea tree oil for disinfecting and 5 drops of lemon oil for a good scent. The shampoo should have a pleasant, slightly thick consistency. Use this shampoo as you would use regular shampoo.

Scabies mites are generally found on the skin. For this, too, Veronika Seher has developed an effective recipe. This neem pesticide is even pleasantly scented.

### Neem pesticide for mites and lice

*10 ml xanthan*
*75 ml distilled water*
*25 ml neem leaf tincture*
*10 drops Paraben K*

Add the xanthan to the water and stir until a thick gel is formed. Now mix the neem leaf tincture into the gel and preserve it with Paraben K. Use the pesticide on your entire body.

## NEEM FOR MOSQUITO BITES

Because mosquitoes that annoy us during the summer or while we're on vacations are also deterred by neem ingredients, we suggest two repellents made with neem oil: a simple one that is easily produced, and a more elaborate one that contains additional essential ingredients.

Repellents are used to repel insects without harming them. If the mosquitoes have already attacked you, the antiseptic and infection fighting characteristics of neem are valuable. The ingredients from the neem leaves are worked into a gel with the aid of an alcoholic extract, which you can then apply to the insect bites.

## Quick repellent

*100 g coconut oil*
*2 g neem oil*
*approximately 20 drops lavender oil (Lavandula angustifolia)*
*approximately 20 drops palmarosa oil*

Slightly heat the solid coconut oil in a water bath until it is liquid. Mix in the neem oil, and let the mixture cool. Then add the essential oils if you wish. Because this mixture is greasy, we recommend that you apply it only to exposed skin.

## Cremaba-based neem repellent

*20 drops tomato green aroma*
*10 drops eucalyptus oil (E. citriodora)*
*10 drops palmarosa*
*5 ml neem leaf tincture*
*50 g cremaba*
*20 ml distilled water*
*10 drops Paraben K*

Mix the essential oils and the neem leaf tincture with the cremaba, then add the water. Stir thoroughly and preserve with Paraben K. Cremaba is a cream that you can obtain in many of the stores listed in the resources section.

Tomato green is a synthetic product that, in contrast to its organic counterpart, does not contain the toxic solanin. It smells like tomato leaves. (The tomato plant is also said to have repelling effects on mosquitoes.)

The neem leaf tincture in the following recipes is produced using neem leaves and alcohol:

## Neem leaf tincture

*50 g neem leaves*
*100 ml alcohol (140 proof)*

Crush or grind the neem leaves, then add the alcohol. Let stand for a week at most and then filter.

## Cooling mosquito gel with neem

*20 drops neem leaf tincture*
*10 ml rose water*
*20 drops menthol*
*1 drop strawflower oil (Helichrysum italicum)*
*5 ml xanthan*
*30 ml distilled water*
*5 ml mild dishwashing liquid*

Combine the neem leaf tincture with the rose water, then add the menthol and the strawflower oil. Now add the xanthan and stir the mass until it thickens. Finally, add the water and the dishwashing liquid, and stir everything thoroughly.

Apply the gel on the mosquito bite as soon as possible. The strawflower oil causes the swelling to go down quickly and complements the cooling effect of the menthol. The gel can also provide relief for wasp and bee bites; however, if you have a reaction, you should also see a doctor after having been bitten because of the danger of allergies.

### Neem mosquito gel with tea tree oil

*10 drops tea tree oil*
*1 drop strawflower oil*
*5 ml xanthan*
*30 ml distilled water*
*10 ml rose water*
*20 drops neem leaf tincture*
*5 ml mild dishwashing liquid*

Mix the tea oil and the strawflower oil with the xanthan until the mass is free of clumps. Then add the water, the rose water, and the neem leaf tincture. To mix the water and oil, add the dishwashing liquid.

This gel can be used like the cooling mosquito gel but is milder and especially well suited for children.

## NOT FOR DRINKING: NEEM TEA

Neem tea is an excellent starting material for cosmetics as well as for the treatment of parasites. But even though people in some countries do drink it, the tea is not entirely suited for internal application because, in my opinion, at present, too little scientific evidence about the effects of the neem ingredients exists.

Neem may become toxic if ingested in large quantities. One study of the effects of neem oil on children indicated the development of a disease somewhat like Reye's syndrome. This may have been caused by outside contaminants rather than by neem, but some observers believe that internal consumption (as with tea) should be undertaken with great caution until its toxicity levels have been further studied.

Neem's pharmacological effects have rarely been studied in controlled environments. However, neem has never been reported to have an adverse effect when used topically or for dental uses.

# COSMETICS 4

In India neem has been used in cosmetics for a long time. Neem products are used in the production of body products of all sorts, for example, in soaps, skin lotions, nail oils, and creams. You can now find several neem cosmetics in health food and alternative stores in Europe and the United States. In my suggested recipes for daily hygiene and beauty care, I use cold-pressed neem oil.

## NEEM FOR THE FACE

### Skin care cream

First the so-called fat phase is produced from which you make a cream by adding water.

#### *Fat phase (60 ml)*
*15 g thick moisturizing cream*
*15 ml almond oil*
*5 ml neem oil*
*10 ml avocado or hazelnut oil*
*5 g cocoa butter*
*10 g shea butter*

Place all ingredients into a heat-resistant pot and slowly melt them at a low temperature (up to seventy degrees Celsius) while stirring constantly. For the production of the final cream, take off 10 milliliters. The remainder is kept in a reclosable container, for example, a jam jar, in the refrigerator. In this manner, it can be kept for up to four months.

### Ready cream (30–35 g)
*10 ml fat phase*
*20–25 ml distilled water*

At about sixty degrees Celsius, add the water to the fat phase (never the other way around) while stirring constantly. Pour the mixture into a reclosable container and shake it thoroughly. The base cream is ready. Once the cream has cooled to lukewarm, mix in the following preservatives. This unique neem cream lasts for about three months.

### Ingredients for 30–35 ml cream
*3 drops Alpha-bisabolol*
*1 pinch allantoin*
*5 drops natural vitamin E*
*4 drops Paraben K*
*approximately 3–5 drops perfume oil of your choice*

## Neem facial wash

This mild facial wash is slightly disinfecting and, because of the hamamelis water, contracting. Aloe vera gives moisture, and fluid lecithin acts as a mild emulsifier. The meristem extract is obtained from embryonic plant cells and acts as a free-radical catcher; that is, it renders aggressive and carcinogenic substances harmless.

### Phase A
*90 ml rose water*
*5 ml aloe vera gel*

### Phase B

*25 drops neem oil*
*5 ml fluid lecithin*
*approximately 5–10 drops perfume oil of your choice*

Mix the ingredients of phase A. Mix the ingredients of phase B together and then add to phase A while stirring constantly. Stir the entire mass.

This facial wash lasts six to eight weeks. For an effectiveness of six months, you may add 20 drops of Paraben K. Because neem oil will collect at the bottom of the container after a while, it is wise to shake the facial wash before each use. Apply the facial wash with a cotton swab to your pre-washed face.

## NEEM FOR HAIR AND NAILS

### Neem shampoo

*30 ml Face-Tensid*
*30 ml distilled water*
*7–8 ml Rewoderm HT*
*1 measuring spoon nuratin*
*1 measuring spoon fragrance-free conditioner*
*1 g neem oil*
*10 drops D-Panthenol*
*approximately 10–15 drops perfume oil*
  *of your choice*
*20 drops Paraben K*

Mix the Face-Tensid with the water. Then gradually add the Rewoderm until the mass acquires the desired shampoo consistency. Then add the nuratin, conditioner, neem oil, D-Panthenol, and a perfume oil of your choice. Nuratin is an albumin hydrolysis from wheat that makes hair shiny. With the addition of Paraben K, this shampoo lasts for about six months.

## Neem hair water

### Phase A

*3 ml poison ivy extract*
*10 g neem leaves (crushed)*
*80 ml lukewarm water*

### Phase B

*5 drops natural vitamin E*
*5-10 ml alcohol (180 proof) or cosmetic hair water*
*5 ml mild dishwashing liquid*
*3 drops essential oil (tea tree oil or rosemary oil)*

Add the poison ivy extract and the neem leaves to the lukewarm water. Let the mixture sit for two hours and then filter it. This is phase A.

For phase B mix the vitamin E into the alcohol, and while stirring constantly, add the dishwashing liquid. Then mix in the essential oils. Slowly mix phase B with phase A.

This hair water lasts about eight weeks. With the addition of thirteen drops of Paraben, its effectiveness is extended to six months.

It is best to pour the hair water into a pipette bottle for application on the scalp. Always shake the hair water before use. Then spread one to two milliliters of the hair water on your scalp and massage in with your finger tips.

## Nail care oil

*10 drops neem oil*
*10 g oil (for example hazelnut oil or haw seed oil)*
*3 drops Face-Tensid*
*10 drops nuratin*

Simply mix all ingredients together and put into an empty lip gloss container or a small reclosable bottle. This nail oil should be applied to the nails on a regular basis, preferably daily.

## NEEM FOR THE BODY

### Liquid neem soap

> *40 ml water*
> *35 ml Face-Tensid*
> *5 ml Sanfteen*
> *2–3 ml Rewoderm HT*
> *1 g neem oil*
> *approximately 8–12 drops perfume oil of your choice*
> *20 drops Paraben K*

Mix the water with the Face-Tensid and the Sanfteen. Then slowly mix in the Rewoderm until the mixture reaches the desired soap consistency. Next add the neem oil and the perfume oil of your choice. Mix everything thoroughly and pour into a soap dispenser. When preserved with Paraben K, this soap lasts five to six months.

### Neem bath oil

> *5 g algae oil*
> *3 g neem oil*
> *70 ml fatty oil of your choice (for example almond or avocado oil)*
> *13 ml mulsifan*
> *possibly 10 ml perfume oil or 5 ml essential oil*

All ingredients are mixed with one another; no heating is necessary. Mulsifan serves as the emulsifier for the bath oil. About one to two tablespoons of this mixture should be added per full tub. This bath oil has excellent moisturizing qualities.

## TOOTH GEL

I have developed a refreshing tooth gel with ground neem bark. For neem bark powder, check the resources section at the end of the book.

Be it shampoo, hair water, soap, or toothpaste— the antibacterial and healthy qualities of neem's ingredients are used in many other health care products as well.

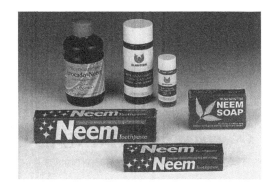

## Tooth gel with neem powder

*1 g stevia powder (sweetener)*
*50 ml distilled or boiled water*
*10 ml betain*
*5 ml xanthan*
*10 ml glycerin*
*3 drops tea tree oil*
*5 drops mint oil*
*12 drops Paraben K*
*5 g neem bark powder*

Dissolve the stevia powder in the water, add betain and xanthan and carefully mix them in. Finally, add the glycerin and the essential oils to the gel, and use the Paraben to preserve it. Sprinkle the neem powder onto the gel and distribute it evenly. Put the gel into an open-ended metal tube and close it.

# Animal Care 5

Because of their usefulness in pest control, neem substances are also valued for animal care. Because our pets probably suffer more from vermin than our plants, we prepared an especially effective mixture for them. With this recipe, you can free your pet of fleas, lice, mites, and other insects.

## Neem animal shampoo

> *4 g neem seeds (ground)*
> *10 drops tea tree oil*
> *100 ml lukewarm water*
> *70 ml Face-Tensid*
> *5 ml fragrance-free conditioner*
> *about 10 ml Rewoderm HT*

The ground neem seeds are mixed with the tea tree oil, which has disinfecting qualities, and the water. Stir frequently, and let the mixture sit for three hours. Then filter it through a sieve, and afterward through a nylon stocking.

Mix the Face-Tensid with the conditioner, which

has an antielectric effect, and add it to the neem solution. In order for the dog shampoo to be easily spread, add about 10 grams of Rewoderm to the mixture. The shampoo should have a slightly thick consistency.

Cats do not like to be bathed. Try spraying them with the raw, watery neem extract using a spray bottle. You can also keep the sleeping area of your pet largely free of pests using neem.

### Bags for dog and cat beds

Place about 50 grams of ground neem seeds in a large handkerchief. If your pets are not particularly sensitive to smell, you can add a few drops of lavender oil or palmarosa oil. Tie the handkerchief, and place the bag in your pet's basket. Of course, you can also place several bags throughout your home in your animal's places.

## ANIMAL FEED

In India, neem has also long been used as an animal and poultry feed. Neem leaves may be helpful in alleviating a copper deficiency from a diet of solely straw and dry fodder. Goats and camels love neem leaves. Quite frequently, they are fed only these in the winter season.

Cattle are fed neem twigs and leaves in small quantities, mixed in with their other feed. Neem residue can also serve as food for cattle. Mixed in small amounts, it is accepted by cattle in spite of its bitter taste. One-tenth to 1 percent mixtures of ground-up neem residue added to regular food prove surprisingly effective against flies: the active ingredients of the neem pass through the intestines of the animals and, in their excrement, prevent further development of the flies' larvae.

Chickens can digest neem oil, as well. The fatty acid composition of the oil makes it a rich source of long chain fatty acids. This oil can be added to poultry rations.

# A NATURAL PESTICIDE 6

## Neem against Grasshopper Plagues

The impressive effects of neem against insects were first observed with desert grasshoppers. It is thus no surprise that scientists soon attempted to control this plague with neem extracts. During their research, the scientists found that the hormones of these insects are disrupted by neem in a very particular way. This is because there is a hormonal shift before the grasshoppers get ready for the attack.

Desert grasshoppers usually live alone and pose no threat to agriculture. Only when too many of them meet and their territory decreases in size does their transformation from harmless hopper to dangerous insect take place.

If at this point in time they are forced to take in neem ingredients from sprayed plants, they fairly soon transform into their original harmless form. The insects then can no longer group together into their dangerous swarms since the hormones that direct behavioral changes are disturbed.

But in nature, it usually does not go this far: the dangerous traveling grasshopper or desert grasshopper avoids the neem

When desert grasshoppers as larvae are sprayed with neem oil, their antennas, legs, and wings become crippled as can be seen with this grasshopper. The insects are no longer able to move and can no longer cause damage.

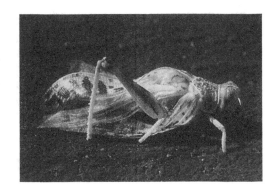

tree. It even has its own mouth apparatus to identify the tree's active ingredients.

The grasshoppers not only recognize the neem tree but also the plants that have been sprayed with neem extracts. If presented with the choice of snacking on these plants or of starvation, the insects choose starvation. Up to two weeks after the treatment, the grasshoppers are able to detect the neem extracts, regardless of climatic conditions. Only after this time will the plants be tasty to them again.

For an effective grasshopper treatment, it is important to prevent dangerous swarms from the outset. For this reason, early alert services are currently monitoring the grasshopper situation in Africa. At the first indication of a possible catastrophe, the threat of a grasshopper plague is supposed to be prevented with neem by averting the congregation of the insects.

## NEEM AGAINST BIRCH LEAF MINERS

A plant health professor in Canandaigua, New York, Dan Marion, Ph.D., has for several years looked for earth-friendly methods to control birch leaf miners, tiny wasps that greatly affect birch trees in the Midwest and Northeast of the United States. The wasps turn birches into brown-leafed skeleton trees. Marion has had good success in controlling these pests by making direct injections of neem into the bases of the trees.

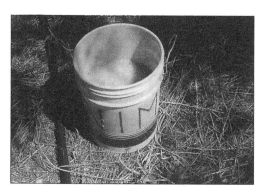

After the neem seed extract is filtered off, a slightly milky spray remains, which reliably protects your plants from hungry insects.

Working in cooperation with the U.S. Department of Agriculture in Beltsville, Maryland, Dr. Marion and his students first tested the extract in spray form. They suppressed 80 to 85 percent of the leaf miners by spraying the foliage with a 1 percent neem solution just after the small insects had deposited their eggs.

Their second experiment consisted of injecting the solution directly into the trees' bases in early May, just as the leaf miners were depositing their eggs in the trees. For comparison, two chemical pesticides normally used for this problem were injected into other trees, and a control group of trees was treated with only water. The water-treated trees became infested with an enormous number of leaf miners—160 adult wasps per 100 grams of leaves. The neem-treated trees had only 3 adult wasps per 100 grams, approximately the same rate as the trees treated with chemicals. The researchers achieved more control through the internal application than by spraying.

Because the root injection system was designed for professional application, a commercial injection system is currently being tested that may be available in the near future.

## NEEM'S WEAPONS

Plants have developed weapons to defend themselves against their enemies. They sting with thorns, release burning poisons upon touch, or produce special substances that keep them from falling prey to their enemies.

The neem tree guards itself against insects that would like only too much to snack on its different parts, with substances they are sensitive to. As a provider of this natural insecticide, it, of course, deserves special appreciation: its products offer numerous possibilities for application and are extremely effective.

Its biologically active ingredients are found in all parts of the tree, but especially in the leaves, and in a highly concentrated form in the seeds. Crushed leaves or ground-up seeds can, with the help of water, alcohol, or solvents, be converted into an effective insecticide. Recipes for the production of a water-based neem spray can be found at the end of this chapter.

The extracts contain a mixture of about forty different ingredients. The exact breakdown of these ingredients varies depending on the precise means of production. Aside from azadirachtin, which is the most important ingredient, there are three more highly active combinations— salannin, meliantropin, and nimbin or nimbidin. Each of these has one or more specific functions in the fight against insects. The remaining, less active ingredients of the tree, whose structures are by now almost completely known, complement this insecticide cocktail. The ingredients complement and amplify one another to produce a highly potent mixture.

In the past decade entomologists have tested neem substances on more than four hundred different kinds of insects. Scientists researched the effects of neem on several mites, nematodes, fungi, bacteria, and various viruses. According to their results, neem concentrations of less than one-tenth part per million in the mixtures would suffice for effective protection against some insects. This is equivalent to 0.00001 percent, approximately one teaspoon of neem in 4,000 liters of water. Some insects start to avoid otherwise attractive plants even with such minute traces of neem.

In laboratory experiments, American scientists observed the

effects of neem on one of the most voracious garden pests of the United States, the Japanese beetle. The greedy beetles were offered a variety of foods and had to decide between life and death. Their favorite food, the leaves of soybean plants, was offered to them, but one-half of the leaves had been sprayed with neem. Within forty-eight hours, they ate the neem-free leaves while not touching those that had been sprayed. The beetles died of starvation before they ate even the smallest part of one of the leaves treated with neem.

Currently, the National Arboretum in Washington, D.C. is using neem to treat various insect infestations on their huge plant collection.

## ETERNAL YOUTH

But neem cannot spoil the appetites of all insects this easily. If they do eat plant material treated with neem, the neem substances then get inside the body of the insect and drastically intervene in the organism's functions. Normal growth is delayed, and problems in development can even result in infertility.

The metabolisms of insects are controlled by a sensitive hormonal system, which is easily disrupted by certain neem substances. Azadirachtin especially has an effect. Its structure resembles the hormone ecdysone, which promotes molting and maturation in insects.

After the insect breaks out of the egg, the development of the young creature, accompanied by repeated shedding, begins. The larvae grow very quickly, and the skin soon becomes too tight. Under the influence of the shedding hormone, a larger, new skin forms under the old one, which is also eventually shed. Among some insects, for example bedbugs and lice, this process is repeated several times. They become closer in appearance to the mature animal, until the mature, fertile animal appears after the last shedding.

Among other insects, for example flies, mosquitoes, and fleas, the full-grown larvae turn into a cocoon. The complete transformation to a mature insect happens in one developmental step. This metamorphosis is also governed by ecdysone.

The ecdysone production is reduced according to azadirachtin concentration, so that at some point no further shedding is possible. The synthesis and release of the real hormone is eventually concluded, and, as a result, further steps in development never occur. If they do not die quickly, the larvae remain for some time as "eternally young" in their most recent stage of development.

## No Resistance

A serious problem that regularly happens with the use of a synthetic insecticide is increasing resistance. Numerous insects become tolerant to formerly highly effective insecticides. A typical example of this is the anopheles mosquito, which transmits malaria to humans. Because of genetic changes brought about by long-term exposure to the insecticide DDT, it has acquired complete immunity to this substance.

Among each type of insect, mutations exist, and if some of these mutations, because of their different genetic makeup, are less sensitive to an insecticide, they will survive the treatment and continue to procreate. A new generation is born, all immune to the insecticide. New populations occur within a short period, and these immune insects will be harder to fight.

Resistance to insecticides is acquired more quickly if only one part in the metabolism of the organisms is affected. The fewer points of action an insecticide has, the greater the probability that the insects will be unaffected. Thus, failure of synthetic chemical products that often contain only one active ingredient is inherent.

The complex mixture of active ingredients in neem, on the other hand, prevents the rapid acquisition of immunity. Several studies whose goal it was to provoke resistance against neem among various insects have proven this fact. For example, cabbage moths in the 35th following generation reacted the same as the parent generation to neem. While a gradual building of resistance with the use of pure azadirachtin would be possible, it does not seem likely.

Certain neem ingredients that take away the vitality of fertile insects play a role in this process. Neem apparently causes fertile insects to enter a state of confusion: they fly less or not at all, and thus do not find partners. The females lay no or significantly fewer eggs.

By this means, the procreation of resistant animals becomes highly unlikely, and the cycle of acquired resistance is stopped at the core. With careful application of the natural combination of active ingredients, scientists predict neem to be effective for a long time.

## NEEM AND FLIES

Flies can become an enormous plague for humans and animals and can become a serious danger if they transmit infectious diseases. The poor countries of the globe, with mostly tropical climates, have invasions of flies that land on humans and animals and are nearly impossible to get rid of.

Some of these flies earlier may have walked on cadavers or excrement, and traces of these (invisible to the human eye) still stick to their legs. With this, bacteria as well as viruses are transported, causing bursitis as well as infectious diseases. Not only humans but also many animals fall victim to diseases transmitted in this way. Since the connection between flies, insufficient hygiene, and such infections is known, many countries of the Third World use chemical synthetic insecticides to fight flies.

Because neem exhibits a variety of effects against harmful insects, these trees might also be able to play a part in the fight against flies. For his doctoral dissertation, the biologist Max Ondongo from Brazzaville in the Congo is researching how flies can be fought and decimated using neem ingredients. At the Institute for Applied Biology at the University of Bonn, he works with two types of flies, the golden fly *(Lucilia cuprina)* and the shin fly *(Stomoxys calcitrans).*

The golden fly does not bring honor to its name. In its home, Australia and South Africa, it is a feared parasite of sheep. The females lay their eggs on the noses of the animals, inside their genital openings, and on parts of their skin soiled with urine and excrement. The maturing maggots immediately work their way inside the skin of the sheep and cause sensitive wounds. With special enzymes, they are able to actually dissolve the tissue of the sheep in these areas.

Up to five hundred larvae parasites exist at the same time on one sheep, and a single fly can lay up to 140 eggs. At first, the larvae place the sheep under considerable duress. The maggot invasions are usually followed by infections that accompany a high fever. In many cases, the sheep die of these infections.

Laboratory experiments in Bonn show that diluted neem extracts significantly reduce the fertility of the female flies. Often the treated flies do not lay any eggs at all. Moreover, it has been shown that the diluted extract irreversibly damages their ability to fly. The flies are no longer even able to rise into the air.

Neem oil has drastic effects on the eggs: not a single larvae emerges from the treated eggs. Young larvae react extremely quickly to the oil; they die within three hours.

Of course, these are laboratory results that cannot immediately be transferred to the real world. Maybe the effect of neem on the egg or the larvae will not be the same. Furthermore, female flies have to be encouraged to eat neem by using bait. Thus far, sugar baits have been successful in the laboratory.

The second type of fly, the shin fly, also reacts strongly to neem's ingredients. Male as well as female flies scrape the skin of their victims and drink their blood. Usually animals are attacked by the hungry flies; in some cases, they have attacked humans as well. Here too, diseases are transmitted from the flies during their meal. The first experiments with neem on shin flies are promising.

But the golden fly and the shin fly are only two examples. Ondongo hopes to fight a number of different types of flies with neem in his home country. He has a very concrete idea of how this is to come about: the key to this lies with toilets.

At most, 30 percent of the Congolese have modern flush toilets that are connected to a sewage system. The remaining part of the population uses a hole under the house for the disposal of excrement. The hole, relatively large, generally occupies an area of about three to four square meters and is about ten meters deep.

About every three years, the smelly contents of this hole are pumped off. In the meantime, the hole serves as a playground for the meatfly and other vermin. Millions of larvae live in the feces; they later swarm out through the toilet opening as infection-transmitting flies.

With neem extracts, it would be possible to pour diluted neem solution or neem oil into the hole. The maturing meatfly could be treated with neem bait. By this means, it should be possible to drastically reduce the population density of flies in the Congo.

But things have not progressed that far yet. Ondongo is currently collecting further data to support his strategy. He then hopes that politicians in his home country might be convinced of the idea of fighting flies with neem. Without their political and financial support, the realization of this idea would be impossible.

So far, officials still place their trust in chemicals. Maybe this is because they do not yet know about the possibilities of application of the neem tree. Even though the neem tree could grow in the Congo, it is still largely unknown there.

## NEEM AS PLANT PROTECTOR

"Eat or be eaten" is one of nature's mottoes. Yet not all insects are plant eaters. Many are thieves or parasites, living off organisms living on plants. With their large appetite, they ensure a moderate number of plant-eating insects.

For example, the plant louse that lives on and off plants has a number of natural enemies. Probably the most well known is the ladybug. With its immense appetite even as a larvae it eats about four hundred of these organisms. And after it breaks out of its cocoon, the mature beetle also prefers to live off these small insects. Other insects, such as the running beetle, in the span of one day eat up to ten caterpillars or larvae of harmful butterflies or beetles, and many birds also ingest a number of insects.

The fighting of plant pests with synthetic chemical insecticides rigorously alters this natural balance. Their active ingredients do not differentiate between "useful" and "harmful." They often also affect "good" animals that perform helpful services in plant protection; these "good" creatures deserve our care.

Especially in this regard, neem is generally ahead of the game: only sucking and biting animals that live directly off plant materials are seriously harmed by neem products' active ingredients.

However, this opinion has changed slightly according to a study performed at the Washington State University and reported in early 1998. That study indicated that spraying with neem does toxic damage to ladybugs, helpful insects that feed upon aphids, scale, and other pests. Researchers Julie Banken and John Stark, Ph.D., tested neem to evaluate its entire range of potential exposure and effects. They discovered that the neem sprays sterilized or greatly reduced the egg-laying of adult ladybugs and killed 100 percent of younger larval ladybugs within ten days of treatment.

## No Fear from Neem

Neem remains completely harmless for thieving useful insects, for example some types of wasps. The concentrations in the insects are mostly too small to have effects on those that eat them. Professor Schmutterer, however, speculates that aside from their food procuring differences, metabolic differences also explain neem's varying effects.

Butterflies and bees, creatures that merely nip on nectar and pollen, do not take in significant amounts of neem. The possible adverse effects of neem on such useful insects is something that scientific studies always keep an eye out for.

So far, however, negative results for smaller bee populations have only been observed in experiments in which strong neem solutions were applied to flowering plants repeatedly. The returning working bees with the collected pollen and nectar were also fed neem ingredients that retarded development of the younger bees. These neem treatments did not have any effect on medium- to large-size bee populations.

The final evidence that neem is not threatening for bees, however, has yet to be established. The careful application of neem extracts is important. Treat especially your flowering plants with the low doses of neem extracts recommended here and do not exceed the recommended frequency of application. If possible, do not spray the flowering parts. Then you will produce the best results.

Studies with earthworms showed that neem can even have positive effects on some useful insects. In greenhouses the worms showed increasing growth rates if the soil was mixed with neem leaves or neem seeds. While in the outdoors, the worm population did not increase, each individual worm developed better in neem-treated than in regular soil.

Scientists in Hawaii discovered a wonderful example of the gentleness of neem substances in the biological regulation of insects. In Hawaii, fruit flies that each year cause great damage in the fruit plantations were tested for their sensitivity to neem. While the fruits were ripening on the trees, the young insects in cocoons were developing into the mature nuisances they would become in the soil. By spraying the soil with a water-based neem solution, the maturing and swarming of the flies could be completely stopped.

But that was not all: a certain type of ichneumon that grows as a parasite in these fruit fly cocoons and is used for biological insect reduction in the plantations proved to be neem resistant. A neem concentration sufficient for the insect allowed the ichneumon to continue their development unaffected in growth as well as in reproduction.

An insect weakened by neem can continue to serve as food for wasps. In contrast, an intervention with a synthetic insecticide would have wiped out all fruit fly larvae.

*NOTE: In the United States, two neem products—neem oil and neem oil, clarified hydrophobic—have recently been approved as pesticide active ingredients by the Office of Pesticide Programs of the United States Environmental Protection Agency.*

## Neem Oil in the Household

In India stored grain reserves are traditionally protected against parasites for three to six months by adding neem leaves. Neem oil has proven to be especially effective at deterring legume parasites. Although neem oil's application on a large scale is still rare, it is used in private households or for seeds that are intended for sowing.

Neem oil has a deterring odor to many insects, which certainly facilitates its storage. Neem oil seems to have a repelling or deterring action against mosquitoes; it has been used successfully for quite some time in mosquito-deterring lotions.

Storage parasites have been on the rise in our apartments over the past few years, partly because of the increase of untreated bio-products and stored pet food. Aside from grain moths, clothes moths also cause considerable damage. You can drive out these annoying roommates with the following recipe:

### Furniture polish

*10 g carnauba wax*
*5 g thick moisturizing cream*
*25 g coconut oil*
*5 g neem oil*
*55 ml hot water*
*1 g each of palmarosa, lavender, cedar, citronella oil*
*2.5 g mild dishwashing liquid*

Melt the carnauba wax, moisturizing cream, coconut oil, and neem oil in a pot or heat-resistant container at a temperature of about eighty degrees Celsius. Mix in water of the same temperature, and let the mixture cool down. Mix the oils with the dishwashing liquid, and then mix them with the grease mixture. Put the polish into a container with a lid. Apply with a soft rag and repolish if necessary.

## Neem as Moth Protection

You can protect expensive rugs and coats from deterioration by spraying them with a watery neem solution. Be careful since light clothing is prone to staining during this treatment. With repeated treatment, the hungry and destructive larvae of the clothes moths will die.

Clothes moths are also affected by a mixture of essential oils and neem oil. The oils can be applied on neem leaves as well as on neem seed flour. Put the material into a bag and place in the closet.

### Moth repellent on neem leaves

*20 drops lavender oil*
*10 drops cedar wood oil*
*10 drops citronella oil*
*50 g neem leaves*

Drip the oils onto the neem leaves and place them in a cotton bag.

### Moth repellent on neem flour

*20 drops lavender oil*
*10 drops stone pine oil*
*10 drops pine oil*
*50 g neem seeds (ground)*

Drip the essential oils on the neem flour and put into a cotton bag.

## Neem as Wood Protection

Even wood pests can be kept away using neem. Outdoors you can prepare wood with the following oil mixture:

*5 g bee's wax*
*40 g turpentine*
*37 g linseed oil*
*15 g neem oil*
*3 g tea tree oil*

Melt the wax and add the turpentine and oils. Apply the mixture onto the wood with a paintbrush or a cotton rag. You may wish to make a small cut into the wood in order to increase absorption of the mixture. Allow some time for the mixture to be absorbed since it is very oily. Repeat the process if necessary. This treatment is especially well suited for garden furniture and bird feeders.

## Recipes for the Treatment of Plants

Before we explore the recipes for the treatment of plant insects of all sorts, here's one small tip for treatment with neem: be patient! Compared with chemical means, the insects do not fall off the leaves all at once after a neem treatment. They may survive for up to another two weeks on the plant. However, they are merely vegetating and are no longer causing any damage to the plant.

This plant care mixture can be used for light to medium infestations and for protection against further damage through eating; it also can serve to strengthen the plant. This recipe can be produced in larger amounts as long as the proportions are kept the same:

### Plant care mixture with neem

*25 g neem seeds (ground)*
*0.5 l lukewarm water*

Place the ground neem seeds in a container. Pour the water over them, mix well, and leave the mixture for up to four hours. Empty the broth through a sieve and then filter it through a nylon stocking. If there are still solid particles in the solution, filter it again.

Carefully wring the remaining broth out of the stocking. A spray that you can apply to your plants either with a spray-bottle or with a paintbrush is now ready. For larger areas, use professional neem spray products available in some garden stores.

The plants should be treated every ten days until they have been largely freed of insects. While applying the treatment, make sure to apply the solution to the undersides of the leaves as well. Often sucking and biting insects hide there and can cause great damage.

Today, time is money for many people. The preparation of this solution may cause some to forgo the treatment. For this reason, we advocate for the production of a ready-made plant care mixture in which the neem ingredients are preserved and remain effective for longer. We hope that such a product will be available soon. It will then probably be offered in the stores listed in the resources section.

## Neem against Garden Mites

Neem seems to have strong deterring effects on many types of mites. While you cannot make the garden mites (also called Grasor fall mites) extinct by means of neem, you can contain them. You should water your lawn with the plant care mixture. For garden mites and their larvae, this treatment is extremely unpleasant.

However, new creatures from a related area will enter your garden again. That is why you should make life more difficult for these insects by taking certain precautions: remove composting piles since mites like to settle in a rotting and wet environment. You should not leave cut grass lying on the ground since the hungry mite larvae love it. When you remove cut grass, you remove a majority of the larvae at the same time.

If you suspect garden mites, you should change your clothes after working in the garden and perhaps take a shower.

You can easily find out whether you have fall mites in your garden, or whether any other parasites have nested there. Slowly drag a white linen cloth over the grass on a warm afternoon. The mite larvae will cling to the cloth and run around on it. It will be easy for you to spot them against the light background. If you want to be completely sure whether the tiny red dots are garden mites, place some of the creatures into a glass tube and send them to the parasitic department of the nearest university for identification.

Regardless whether the test comes back positive or negative, you can get rid of a number of insects with neem extract. Neem can also protect your pet from insects. You can apply the water-based neem solution with a spray bottle on your dog and on your cat (if she does not run away). The sour neem odor will cause mites, ticks, and fleas to disappear.

You can even spread neem solution on your own skin. If you decide to treat yourself, you should first place a drop of the solution on a small area of your skin to test whether you are allergic. After all, allergies are always possible, especially with natural products.

## NEEM AGAINST PERNICIOUS INSECTS

For insects such as lice and others, here is another recipe. Added fluid lecithin quickens the effectiveness of neem because of its content of soy oil: the oil clogs the breathing passages of the insects and causes them to suffocate. The essential oil (lavender or geranium oil) spreads a scent repulsive to insects. Lecithin and tea tree oil are also effective against mildew. The additional pinch of vitamin E protects the neem ingredients against quick dissolution by oxygen.

### Plant protection mixture with neem

*12 g (2 heaped tablespoons) neem seeds (ground)*
*5 g fluid lecithin CM*

*5 drops tea tree oil*
*5 drops lavender oil (provence) or geranium oil*
*1 pinch natural vitamin E*
*250 ml lukewarm water*

Thoroughly mix the ground neem seeds in a container with fluid lecithin CM, tea tree oil, and lavender or geranium oil. Then add vitamin E. Once a well-mixed mass has formed, add the water in small amounts.

The mixture should breathe for three hours while being stirred frequently. Then pour it through a kitchen sieve and filter it through a nylon stocking. If there are still solid particles in the solution, filter it through the stocking a second time.

Apply the mixture all over the plant using a paintbrush or a spray bottle. The treatment should be repeated every seven to ten days. This neem solution can be kept in the refrigerator. Through the addition of 20 drops of Paraben K per 100 milliliters of solution, the neem solution will remain effective for fourteen to twenty days.

We are also working on the production of a ready-made solution for these insects in which the neem ingredients have been conserved to retain their effectiveness for longer periods of time. We hope that such a product will be offered in stores soon.

## NEEM AGAINST MILDEW

Recently a new branch of research on the neem tree and its fascinating abilities has developed. After the water-based and alcohol extracts of the neem seeds with their limonoid components were in the foreground of scientific research for years, neem oil with its own—and no less stunning—qualities has now become more prominent.

Scientists at the University of Giessen have been testing the effectiveness of cold-pressed neem oil against mildew on different plants with much success. This fungi is not only the enemy of all rose gardeners, it also annually causes great economic damage in the planting of, for example, grapes and cucumbers. Certain oils cause an immunization of the plant against this disease. Neem oil with its particular ingredients is a fungicide.

Scientific knowledge is available about the treatment of so-called real mildew on cucumbers and apples. It is highly probable that neem is effective against mildew on other fruit trees and raspberries, but this has yet to be scientifically proven.

For this application, neem oil first has to be strongly diluted with water. The pure oil causes not only the bad insects but also the useful insects to die; furthermore, it clogs up the pores of the plants, making them prone to suffocation. The alkaline effects of the concentrated oil can also lead to damage in the plant tissue.

Oil and water can only be mixed with the help of an emulsifier. An especially mild emulsifier suited for plant care is obtained from castor oil and carries the name rimulgan. In the course of experiments, sodium hydroxide ($NaHCO_3$), commonly known in the household for curing heartburn and an important component of baking soda, surprisingly proved to be effective in plant protection as well. As an additional component in the emulsion, it amplifies the effects of the oil. Following the motto "Together we are stronger," scientists developed the following recipe as a cure for affected plants as well as a prophylactic for healthy ones:

### Neem oil against mildew

> *5 g lukewarm neem oil (cold-pressed)*
> *2.5–5 g mild dishwashing liquid*
> *2.5 g baking soda*
> *1 l water*

Mix the lukewarm liquid neem oil well with the dishwashing liquid. You can slightly warm the neem oil to about thirty to thirty-five degrees Celsius for easier processing in a water bath. Dissolve the baking soda in the water. While intensively stirring, add the soda solution in small portions to the mixture until a milky emulsion forms.

Before usage, shake the mixture thoroughly. The ready lotion can be applied to the plants with a pump spray bottle or with a soft paintbrush. This treatment should be repeated after ten days.

Neem oil will keep its effectiveness for a long time if it is stored in a dark, cool place (preferably the refrigerator). Another means to extend its life is the immediate preparation of the oil emulsifier mixture as described in the recipe. For individual applications, you then simply measure off the desired amount and  add water and sodium hydroxide.

Scientists at the University of Giessen under the direction of Dr. Bernd Steinhauer tested this mildew treatment successfully not only as a prophylactic, but also against existing mildew. In this highly effective recipe, the various active ingredients amplify one another: in neem oil, the oil components as well as the individual ingredients are active. Sodium hydroxide complements the effects of the oil on mildew, probably by destroying the comfortable environment the fungi enjoy.

## Neem with Systemic Usage

Aside from the application of neem extract on the plant, there is another interesting alternative. In this case, the extract is not applied to the parts of the plant, but is added to the soil by watering or spraying. The ingredients reach the roots of the plants, are absorbed by them, and by means of the water-distributing system of the plant, the xylem, are spread throughout the plant. This procedure is referred to as systemic.

The internal protective effects also prepare growing parts of the plant for their fight against the insects. This treatment only affects those insects that live off the green of the plant, and not, for example, the bees and other useful thieving insects. In addition, a sudden rain cannot simply wash away the effectiveness of the extract.

Unfortunately the treatment is not equally effective in all cases. There are marked differences depending on plant and insect type. The best preconditions for effective use of the systemic treatment are a sufficient concentration, a good absorption of the ingredients, and a good distribution within the plant.

Satisfying results have been observed with wheat, greens, rice, tomatoes, cotton, and chrysanthemum. Strengthened by systemic means, the leaves and stems of the plants remained untouched by typical insects for about ten weeks. While bean plants absorb the main ingredient azadirachtin without problems, this does not happen with the potato plant.

The particular enzymatic activity of a plant determines the time span within which the neem components remain active. That is why further individual tests of plant types are necessary. The acidic content of the soil also has an important effect on the length of the ingredients' effectiveness.

Because of the potential toxic effects on the plants, only extremely well-cleaned extracts should be used in the systemic application. This applies especially to the use of neem oil.

For the successful control of insects, their respective preference for various plant parts is important, since they have to contain neem ingredients in sufficient concentrations. Protection, for example, is not effective with certain kinds of plant louse that only feed off the outermost layer of the plant tissue, the phloem.

# POLITICS 7

## PATENT FIGHT OVER A NATURAL PRODUCT

Because this tree holds so much promise, big corporations have become interested in neem. While companies in the past considered neem researchers to be alternative lunatics, some corporations are now sensing big money in neem. The American firm, W. R. Grace, with global headquarters in Boca Raton, Florida, has already applied for and received several patents on products of the neem tree. The company has been making headlines.

A patent on a plant protection product in which the main ingredient of neem was especially long lived has attracted criticism of international environmental and natural organizations. They fear (and not without reason) that W. R. Grace will make big money with the neem products while the farmers that cultivate neem trees will receive little.

The Foundation on Economic Trends, a scientific watchdog group, believes this patent will force Indian farmers to pay top rupee for a substance that used to be almost free. Currently, more than two hundred organizations from thirty-seven nations have mounted a legal challenge in the U.S. Patent and Trademark office against W. R. Grace's patent. Jeremy Rifkin, president of the Foundation on Economic Trends, has called this "genetic colonialism." His group has organized the above coalition.

This type of problem has occurred repeatedly in the past. Poor countries of the Third World are being exploited by wealthy industrial nations as a cheap source for raw materials. While W. R. Grace is said to currently be paying decent prices for neem seeds, many farmers are already exporting all of their neem seeds to the United States. There remain none for the domestic market. Thus, synthetic chemical insecticides continue to be used. Neem farmers also become dependent on a single company that has the power to dictate prices.

The young neem trade has no TransFair Initiative, as exists, for example, in the coffee trade. TransFair buys coffee for a fair price directly from cooperatives of small coffee farmers and certifies coffees sold under internationally recognized fair trade criteria. The TransFair concept was begun in the Netherlands as Max Havelaar and was renamed in Germany. TransFair USA started in Oakland, California, in 1998. But responsible neem traders are currently trying to diversify their markets and to not buy up all the neem from one country. They also are trying to establish pricing acceptable to all sides.

Most imports of neem products in the United States are from India, Japan, and Germany.

The mentioned patenting, however, would not affect the world market in the respect that neither the neem tree nor its leaves and seeds can (yet) be patented. The patent then merely extends to the special type of processing that is done by W. R. Grace.

## Conflict with the Plant Protective Law

When I wrote this book, no ready-made plant protection products based on neem were for sale. Neem seeds are exported in whole or ground-up form and are offered as raw material for cosmetics, for pest control, and for animal care products. The same goes for neem leaves and neem oil.

After the serious potential dangers of chemical synthetic insecticides and pesticides became clear, a stringent plant protective law was agreed upon. The effects and concentrations of each active ingredient of a plant protection product have to be well known. Such requirements can be met relatively easily with a chemical synthetic product. With a natural product these requirements are nearly impossible. Depending on place of origin, weather, and climate, the components of the ingredients in each plant vary.

Natural products are not well suited for standardization because of their relatively short life span. Among industrial products, neem needs to be standardized and conserved worldwide, as has been done in the United States. While this is less desirable for the environment, it is a necessary requirement for the bureaucracy. The ecological qualities of a natural substance are thus worsened to comply with the requirements for licensing.

# Your Own
# Neem Tree

8

Neem seeds exported to the United States generally do not germinate since they are too old when they arrive. Furthermore, in our latitudes, there are of course climatic problems. A fresh seed can germinate on the windowsill; however, as an exotic species, it seems to follow its own laws. Upon returning from a trip to Venezuela to study the neem project, I had my pockets full of fresh neem seeds capable of germinating. Friends, acquaintances, colleagues, anyone who wanted them received neem seeds to cultivate their own neem trees. Some seeds germinated within two weeks; others did so in a few months. Most seedlings did not grow any more.

In our winter, the daylight time and intensity were probably too short and too low for the exotic plants. Only a few acquaintances' seedlings even grew to be small plants, and my own plant, which I received as a gift at this size, has so far not exceeded its height of one meter. Only one colleague had unexpected success: she reported after only six weeks about a plant that was already twenty-five centimeters high and nervously inquired about how tall this tree would grow. The growth of this plant was probably encouraged by favorable light and temperature conditions.

Germinable neem seeds can only be obtained from the importer (see resources). The importer guarantees the seeds' ability to germinate for about five months if they are kept in the vegetable compartment of a refrigerator. Neem seeds are much more expensive than more available seeds since a greater effort is needed for their quick transport, storage, and delivery.

Almost everyone has received the shoot of some plant as a gift. This is generally a small branch that has to be put in water. Soon the cutting develops its first roots, and the plant is ready to be placed in a pot.

This possibility, in principle, is also available for the neem tree; however, the chances of us finding someone in Western Europe or the United States who owns a neem tree and has a shoot are very small. So far neem trees exist only in the greenhouses of neem researchers and in a few botanical gardens. With luck, this situation will soon change.

# Resources

**Aegis Azaanim Private Limited**
AD-27, 5th St., Anna Nagar, Chennai 600040, India
Tel: 91-44-6282244, Fax: 91-44-6288891 • www.webindia.com/aegis

**Aina Hawaiian Tropical Products**
www.hawaiiantropicals.com

**Ayurvedic Rasayanas Intl.**
P.O. Box 5966, Eugene, OR 97405
Tel: 541-349-8680, Fax: 541-349-0975 • www.ayurveda-herbs.com

**Bahama Neem Links**
www.ajtsc.com/bahama_Links.htm

**Colimex**
Ringstr. 46
D-50996 Köln, Germany
Tel: 49-221-352072, Fax: 49-221-352071

**Desert Essence,** Tea Tree Oil Toothpaste with Neem
Chatsworth, CA 91311
Available through Gaines Nutrition On-line Health Food Store
www.gaines.com

**The House of Mistry,** Manufacturers and Suppliers of Health, Herbal,
and Homeopathic Products
15-17 South End Road, Hampstead Heath, London, NW3 2PT
England
Tel: 44-171-794-0848, Fax: 44-171-431-5695

**Interpet Laboratories,** A neem-based flea bite shampoo
7517 NW 41st St., Coral Springs, FL 33065
Tel: 954-796-8960 • www.proclus.com/interpet/index.html

**Karani Export Corporation**
#1 Dalal Cottage, S.L. Road, Mulund, Bombay 400080, India
Tel: 91 22 5682259/5653570, Fax: 91 22 5653570

**Life's Vigor,** Vitamins, Minerals, and Supplements
P.O. Box 5653, Bakersfield, CA 93388-5653
Tel: 1-800-871-6848 • On-line store at www.lifesvigor.com

**The Neem Association**
1780 Oakhurst Ave., Winter Park, FL 32789
Also on Bahama Neem Links

**Neem Foundation**
www.neemfoundation.org

**Niem-Handel Gerald Moser**
August-Bebel-Str. 45
D-64347 Griesheim, Germany
Tel/Fax: 49-6155-2790 • www.Niem-Handel.de

**Organix's Natural Health Pharmacy**
www.organix.net/organix/neem_oil.htm

**The Original Neem Company**
2711 NW 6th St., Suite B, Gainesville, FL 32609
Tel: 352-375-2663 Fax: 877-891-6336 • www.neemaura.com

**Plasma Power Private Ltd.**, Supplier of Neem oil for control of crop pests
10 Alsa Arcade, B-8 Second Avenue, Anna Nagar, Chennai 600 102
India
Tel/Fax: 91-44-6368609 • www.plasmaneem.com

**Spinnrad GmbH,** A source for ingredients used in recipes in
Chapters 3–6
Am Bugapark 3
45899 Gelsenkirchen, Germany
Tel: 49-209-17-000-0, Fax: 49-209-17-000-40 • www.spinnrad.com